Disclaimer

The publisher and the author are providing this book and its contents on an "as is" basis and make no representations or warranties of any kind with respect to this book or its contents.

Acknowledgements

I want to thank

My sister,
Dr. Diana Pengitore, ND, freelance translator, and American Translator Association (ATA) member, for her expert translation from German to English.

My brother-in-law,
Dr. Frank Pengitore, Ed. D., for his editorial expertise in bringing this publication forth.

Dedication

I dedicate this book to lovers so that they have a foundation for their love and that their relationship endures.

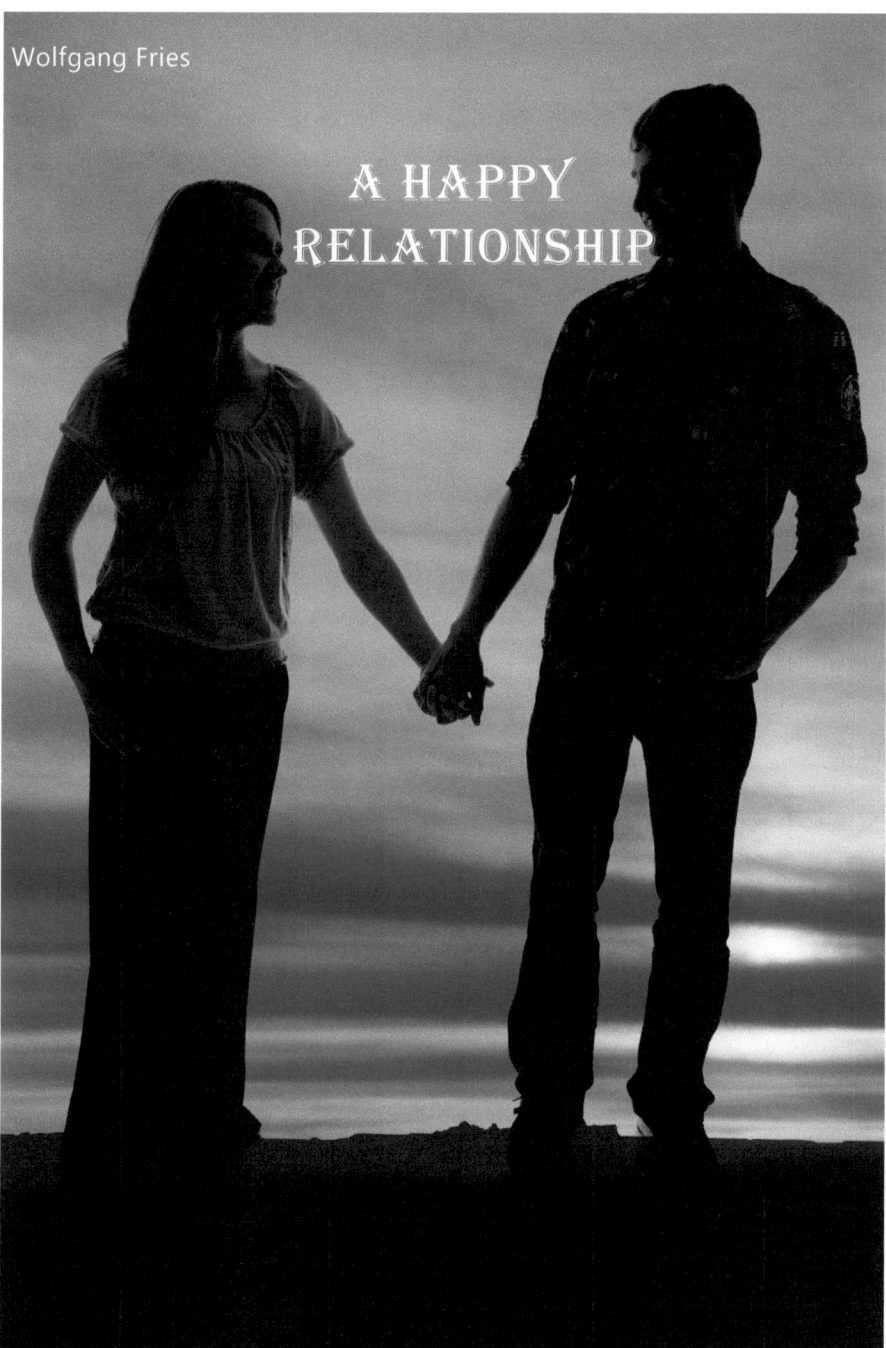

Imprint

Copyrights and clearances
For this publication, literature from L. Ron Hubbard* was utilized. The German book, *Im Leben bestehen - Die Bible des 21sten Jahrhunderts*, has been re-issued as *Philosophie des Lebens - Das Buch der Grundlagen*, from which a part of this book's written texts was taken. All material contained in this book has been approved by the authors whose work has been referenced herein.

Book design and typeset:
Wolfgang Fries
Contact: Friesway@online.de

Translator: Dr. Diana M. Pengitore, ND
Editor: Dr. Frank Pengitore, Ed. D.

Production and publishing:
BoD - Books on Demand, Norderstedt

ISBN: 978-3-7534-7292-8
1. Edition

© 2021 for the content Wolfgang Fries

Bibliografische Information der Deutschen Nationalbibliothek
Die Deutsche Nationalbibliothek verzeichnet diese Publikation in der Deutschen Nationalbibliografie; detaillierte bibliografische Daten sind im Internet über http://dnb.d-nb.de abrufbar.
(The book is listed in the German Nationalbibliografie; detailed information is available at: http://dnb.d-nb.de)

Important note to the reader:

Take great care in reading this text in order not to skip words that you do not understand. If you do not understand a sentence or text, it is because there is a word or words that you did not understand or for which you have a false definition.

In the glossary, an overview of the definitions of the words listed in the book marked by an asterisk* can be found. In order to have a complete understanding of a word, it should be looked up in a good dictionary, including its origin.

Footnotes are used to denote sources and references.

A Happy Relationship

Table of Contents

Introduction 11
The Human Being 12
To Encounter One's Fellow Human Being 13
Love 14
Happiness 15
Principles – The Action's Basics 16
Experiencing Life 16
Persistence - Achieving one's Goals! 17
Setting the Goal 18
Intention is Cause 18
Developing a Strategy 19
The Letter 20
The First Phone Call 20
The Knowledge of Human Nature?! 20
Emotion 25
Love 28
Attractiveness and Character 29
A Few Words About "Life" 31
Exchange Factors 32
The Definition of Reason 32
Responsibility 33
Happiness 35
Happiness and Freedom? 35
Unhappiness 36
The Human's Will Is His Kingdom of Heaven 36
Loyalty, Fidelity and Happiness 38
Do You Know Who Your Friends Are? 41
The Problem Begins in the Head 45
Anatomy* of a Problem 46
Stress 49
War!!! 52
Privacy 54
Getting Something Done! – The Power of the Second Person – ... 55

Getting One's Own Stuff Done..57

Communication – The Key to the World........................58

Having a Conversation...60

The Date...64

The Right One 65

Sex...69

The Desire to Be the Effect...72

Relationship and Logic 74

What Makes the Human Complicated?.........................75

Mature for a Relationship 78

Victim..82

Family 83

A Place in the Heart of the Other 85

The Relationship Fails 86

Still a Few More Trifles 91

Right and Wrong...94

Codex for the Second Dynamic....................................96

Your Rainbow 97

Glossary..99

Sources and References...107

About the Author 109

Other Books 111

Introduction

There are plenty of books on the subject of love and relationship. Everyone is equipped with this feeling called love and would like to experience it, sometimes more and sometimes less. However, one very often gets shipwrecked in this interpersonal* area. The fact is that nobody really seems to truly know anything about the *métier of love. One falls in love and has a relationship – period!

But what is this matter called love? What can one do to ignite love, to maintain it or even eliminate it? What are the rules and laws?

A relationship is based on the individual. There are two individuals who find each other and have a relationship. Consequently, both must have the same attitude to have a healthy relationship. A relationship, therefore, is based on the attitude of the partners.

This book is not only about a relationship with one's partner but also about the attitude that one should have towards a relationship. A relationship is a part of the all-encompassing life, and everyone should realize clearly that the aspects of existence must be brought into harmony to live life well.

The background to this book is my book *Philosophie des Lebens - Das Buch der Grundlagen*, which covers a larger area of existence. It is of no use to be well informed in one area of life when the other areas are very influential and can even destroy one or the other. In order to live a relationship, one should be able to live a life, and this requires some knowledge in today's time and an appropriate attitude!

The Human Being

The human being experiences this world through his mind. If the mind of the individual does not get in order, this world does not get in order.

1. The human is a product of his deeds.
2. He does what he thinks. If he thinks not to do it, he does not do it.
3. The human does not try to do wrong.
4. There are strange actions. Thus, there are strange thoughts*.
5. Since the human tries not to do wrong and still does, there are thoughts that appear stronger than the human wants.
6. Thus, the thought governs the human.
7. Thus, the human is not always the cause of his thoughts.
8. Thus, there is a part in the human that tells him to do wrong.
9. This part confuses him and makes him small, weak and ill.
10. Being ill means doing wrong – no matter what the thought commands. (Millions of years of engineering result in an organism that heals itself, and yet it gets sick.)
11. Thus, the thought organizes matter.
12. And the thought is thought by the being.
13. All thoughts are made of the same, be they good or bad.
14. The bad thought can be resolved. It comes from the bad experiences that one once had and that the human had done before(!).
15. Thus, one again becomes big, strong and healthy.
16. And the human does not have to be human anymore.

Corollary*:
The human changes when he changes his thoughts.
You change the human when you help him change his thoughts.

To Encounter One's Fellow Human Being

How does one get along with one's fellow human beings? There are such things as manners and customs that determine a certain behavior, and which are fixed by rules, be they in writing or not. In fact, these are the moral rules that are supposed to indicate right and wrong.

In short, those who got their driving license in Germany probably are familiar with paragraph one (§1) of the road traffic ordinance. It is actually the case that one interacts with one another within society; hence, this paragraph also can be applied to social interaction among one another as follows:

1. The participation within society requires constant caution and mutual consideration.

2. Every citizen is to behave in such a way that no one is harmed, endangered, hindered or harassed under the circumstances more than is unavoidable.

Remember to treat your fellow human being as a friend - he is not your enemy yet!

In Peacetime

Encounter your fellow human being with a friendly attitude and peaceful intent. Recognize whether he is a help or a burden by his actions.

If he acts in good faith, help him recognize his mistake so that it will be better the next time around.

When the real mistake has been identified, but the goal is not achieved, give him a task that he can do.

If he cannot accomplish the task, then let him go so that he will not bring you bad luck.

A common intention lets individuals form groups as a result of a shared aim. And every group has a leader. This leader should have an intellect superior to all others and guide the group in the best possible way towards a common goal through reason.

If the leader's reason fails, he also fails. He especially can learn.

Every group member has the right to appeal to the leader's reason.

Love

"It is not the person but rather the feeling. One believes that if one loses the person, one loses the feeling. Yet this feeling can always be created anew. There is as much love as there are people."

1. A feeling desired by everyone.
2. Yet, nobody knows where it comes from.
3. It can bring the human being great happiness or great sorrow.
4. The feeling does not come from the being itself but from what makes him into a human being.
5. If the human himself could recognize of what he is made, he could recognize himself and walk the path with love that leads him to great happiness.
6. The feeling is a thought, and it says, "Be together!"
7. It is one's own doing that breaks this feeling.
8. To separate means to protect the other from one's own bad doing to not want to hurt him anymore.
9. A relationship is a choice.
10. This decision is to be for the other. (Note: One can be for or against the other.)
11. The decision is supported by "doing." When one stops doing, the decision withers.
12. Jealousy is supported by the fear of deciding differently. It also can show what the other intends to do.
13. The weak tends to be jealous.
14. The decision of the strong will stand. It is supported by reason.
15. Reason is survival towards pleasure.
16. Pain means to succumb and to not survive in the long run.
17. Communication is the glue of the relationship, and the secret is separation.

Falling in love is easy, but understanding is required to preserve love. By not understanding one another anymore, love falls apart. It is the messed-up mind of the human being that ends understanding!

Happiness

Life gives you a joyful emotion when you help life to live. Ask a woman how she feels after giving birth to her child or a contractor after building a house or when things have been repaired well. All this contributes so life can live! The following are characteristics that can affect happiness:

1. Happiness is the human's highest aspiration.
2. To be happy, the human accepts the loss of freedom because being happy means having what one desires. However, "to have" ends the state of freedom.
3. Thus, the human fell for materialism and the accompanying feeling, thereby creating his own prison.
4. Materialism and feeling can invert*, and the human will be happy again only when he no longer has material possessions or feeling.
5. Thus, we find that by connecting happiness with material things and feeling, that happiness is as fleeting* as these.
6. But there is another form of happiness.
7. Through material things or feeling, the human is in an effect position because material things and feeling act on him.
8. The human can be the cause! He himself can cause things.
9. When the human has a self-fulfilling task that brightens the face of the world in beauty, cultivates* the virtues of the human being and improves the general existence, ensures that things work and are useful or anything else that gives pleasure to his fellow human beings, the human will experience satisfaction and happiness through this activity alone.
10. Thus, we find that through doing the human creates his own happiness.
11. Even the one who has only a little bit of hope in achieving something still has a piece of luck in him; however, when hope fades away, and one has completely given up, then one also has surrendered his luck.
12. The human will fall ill if oppression and counter-intentions have become too great to attain happiness, and he will find ways, obvious or hidden, to get out of existence to escape misfortune.
13. The human can be happy when he is strong and recognizes the basics of symbiosis and reason for himself and lives by them. And so there can be happiness for everyone!

The inability to understand, ignorance, lack of discipline, clumsiness and cowardice are the main factors that stand in the way of happiness.

Happiness means to set something in motion, either towards someone or away from someone; one wants to have things or dispose of them!

But how can one achieve this when one is defeated by one of the above characteristics?

Principles – The Action's Basics

How does the human encounter the events of life? Well, he sees something and acts accordingly. But before he acts, he usually does one thing - he thinks. He sorts his thoughts to do the right thing in a situation without making a mistake that could lead to disadvantages for him.

Certainly, one of the things he will encounter in life is a set of rules established by the state, which presents the right, meaning that if you violate it, you will be punished. Whether the state's law is fair is another matter because right and justice are two different pair of shoes. Thus, the state has its principles. Incidentally, in principles is the word *princi** (princess), and the princess is the one who comes first, at least in the line of succession to the king or queen when there is no male heir in most cases.

Principles: Things that come first, the thought that precedes the action. Thus, one acts according to a principle of a kind and manner because the thought dictates how the person created the thought.

Well, dear friend, you certainly have adopted your own principles from others or learned from experience. Unfortunately, the places of teaching and learning, the public schools, do not give lessons and teach no subject that conveys the principles of life. And yet they are the foundation of life!

So, I sat down and made few notes about it, saw things, formulated it and wrote it down. Maybe you will make these principles yours. In any case, they helped me, and they were the foundations upon which I could rely.

Experiencing Life

To experience existence with all its facets* depends on one thing only, one thought - **"I can!"**

For example, over there is a beautiful girl or a handsome guy who awoke your interest. You see her or him and think, "What can I say? He or she certainly has no interest in me. I do not dare." All of these thoughts tell you, "You cannot!", and all of these thoughts keep you from experiencing your life.

So, think **"I can!"**

Fundamentally, the thought "I can" is the beginning of ability. There is work to be done, such as painting the decking on the roof, building and plastering a wall, creating a workpiece in the company, dealing with a new machine or just writing a letter. You see this work and immediately think, "It is too complicated, too difficult, too daring; I do not understand; another can do it better," and so on. Interestingly, you look only at the thought that wants to tell you that you cannot. You do not even make an attempt to take a look at the matter at hand or think about what is required to face the task.

Think **"I can!"**

Force yourself to hold this thought. The more you hold on to this thought, the more accurately you will look at the matter, and solutions will come to mind. The people around you are only people exactly the same as you with hands and feet and the ability to think.

So, YOU can too!

As a rule, a bit of knowledge, some training and dexterity* is required to be able to approach a matter appropriately. My former master once said the following about the reading of books, "Books are written for people who do not look closely and who do not devise a sufficient solution through their thinking." I personally concur that written words are often just the opinion of a person, usually imagined and not closely observed. Well, I, too, belong among the readers, and I can say that many a book has helped me or that the voice of another has enlightened my mind.

To get something done in the end, it takes intention, and that intention is supported by the thought "I can!" If you lose this thought, you lose your ability and even your life! This world only works because the human dares to take on matters because he says to himself, "I can!"

So think, **"I can"!**

Ability? What is ability other than to disassemble things and to put them back together in a functioning way or to come up with ideas to take the components of the world to create something functional!

Persistence - Achieving One's Goals!

Definition of *persistence:* **A tenacious hold on to an intention to achieve a certain goal.**

Setting the Goal

So, you want to find the right partner. Now the first step would be to imagine exactly how your partner should look and what character he should have. You write this down and add a glued-on picture of how your partner should look. Then, you memorize this in the form of a picture. It may seem strange to you, but this will enable you to create the exact physical event that you have in your head as a picture. Your thought will take shape.

Here are a few examples. It had been a long hot day, and I really wanted a maple walnut ice cream. Well, it was already 8:15 P.M. and the gas station that had this ice cream usually closed right at 8:00 P.M. So, I got into my car and arrived at the gas station just as the attendant was about to close! What a coincidence. She said that she had run out of this flavor of ice cream. I told her that I wanted to take another look. Afterall, the ice box was in the customer area. As luck would have it, there actually was another maple walnut ice cream, the last one of its kind. ☺

On another day, I had the idea of driving through Hamburg* in a high-horse-powered car. Not long thereafter, I was actually in Hamburg driving my boss's car, an Audi Quattro with 200 horsepower.

Remember, at the same moment that you envision your wish, "counter-thoughts*" will arise. Just write them all down and envision your picture once more. Should the "counter-thoughts" return, write these down again and repeat this process as needed. Afterward, burn the paper. The sole purpose of this is because you really want to achieve your goal. You want to move mountains! Believe in yourself and the power of your thoughts. Do not get depressed right away when your desires do not immediately manifest in the material world because if that were the case, you would be God in this universe. Keep in mind that other people also have desires. Functional postulates* are based on the order of magnitude of power. Either a lot of people are against you, or there is someone who just has more power than you!

Intention is Cause

Nothing is caused without intention! When the intention is taken, then nothing more is done. Always stay on the ball. Call, instead of being called. Make an appointment that includes the day and time, and do not say, "Yes, one could do that …"

You can be the game ball in life, or you can play with the ball!

Developing a Strategy

I was a craftsman and kept myself very busy. I did not make time to go out to meet someone. However, since I wanted a relationship, there had to be another way. So, I placed a personal ad in a newspaper and wrote. Nowadays, the whole matter is a bit easier and faster over the Internet. By the way, the people who place a personal ad are interested in getting to know someone.

The people that you meet through an advertisement have enough guts to place an ad. They are able to put aside all the prejudices regarding personal advertisements to do it! You will find that these people are usually open-minded and want to talk to you.

The letter you are writing is the foot in the front door. Use nice-looking stationary with an elegant or romantic theme. Write the letter with a calligraphy pen, a fountain pen with a special nib* for "beautiful writing." Incidentally, the word has its origin from Greek, *kalos* = beautiful and *graphein* = to write. Do not simply write a profile, "25 years old, businessman by profession, 6 feet tall, 176 lbs." NO!!!

Get a picture in which you are photogenic, no macho* pose and not buttoned up, unless you want the lady to think exactly that of you! In this way, I had up to 90% returns. I came to find out later, on the first or second date, that I was one of the few who received a reply. There were women who received up to 80 reply letters to their ad, and often there was only one or two letters that actually sparked interest. The rest were "profiles." By the way, men receive very few or no responses to their ads because women want to be courted.

Keep your letter short to arouse curiosity. Do not introduce yourself because you can do that later on the phone. So, give it your best with your writing and write a perfect letter with no mistakes or cross outs. Use the whole sheet, not just a third. Show that you are making a real effort.

I answered all advertisements that were somewhat interesting, up to 10 pieces per newspaper edition. Keep many options open because you never know what may result.

One thing above all, you must not give up. The more you write, the more will reply to you. There are certainly one or two good paperbacks about writing letters or dealing with the opposite gender. Start reading, and you will find that it makes an impression and is sure to give you one or two good tips.

The Letter

Write what you really want, for example:

Hello!

I want to finally fall in love again and think that this is still possible at 35.

My wish is a partnership in which one is there for the other, enabling us to go through life together without losing oneself.

A relationship is like a flower; it will bloom and flourish when it is taken care of. And that is exactly what I want to do - to create a living space in which this can be.

Best regards,

Wolfgang

P.S. Simply SMS or Letter

The First Phone Call

Be yourself and do not use words that you do not understand. If you can offer a distinguished diction, wait until you realize that the other person also has this at her disposal.

Also mention that you are excited and that you do not know exactly what to talk about. Now it is about breaking the ice. Ask what she would like to know about you. She will ask, and you will answer. Ask her what characteristics her partner should have, what activities she likes, what hobbies she has, where she goes on vacation or would like to go, what club she belongs to, and so forth. Be attentive and listen when she is excited about a topic and be interested.

Honesty and sincerity should always be there. Definition *sincere* : **Expressing the innermost feeling of one's own conviction without disguise.**

The Knowledge of Human Nature?!
"As soon as you deal with a human, you have a problem!"

One should have useful data on this topic because this knowledge alone is decisive in determining your rise or fall! Well, as long as the human does not know exactly what he is, he can have no knowledge of it. Think about it. Do you have a body, or are you a body? If you imagine something, who is looking at this picture? If you are afraid, who feels this fear? It is neither cold nor warm.

The body is a carbon-oxygen machine and runs at 37 degrees Celsius (98.6 degrees Fahrenheit). If we analyze the living and the just deceased body of a human being, we do not find any differences in the chemical analysis of the matter. Every biochemist will confirm that the bones and organs are the same. Yes, even the cell area and the molecules are unchanged if the examination is done promptly. The weight is the same, and even the temperature can be about the same, yet one body lives and the other is dead. It decomposes into its components and turns to earth and dust.

What power, strength and energy must exist to ensure that all matter is shaped and structured in such a way that it forms this living body as we know it? "Everyone has enough measurable electrical current that flows through his organism to light up a 100-watt light bulb".[1]

This is to say that we are dealing with life and that life has its natural laws. The living organism has energy, and this energy is the exact starting point. You sit in a body and provide the energy that the body needs. You are the power and strength that shapes, structures and holds matter together.

Unfortunately, the human being has declined mentally and has reached a low mental state. He thinks more than he observes and concludes. One can imagine the average person like a big bunch of small balloons that are tied together. The incoming communication is like a needle hitting any balloon. One will always get a reaction. The problem with the matter is that this is a stimulus reaction mechanism, and one cannot speak of a factual, sober handling. Thus, the human lives more in his mind than he does observing and clearly recognizing facts.

Example: My girlfriend lost 25 kg* within six months. An acquaintance, who had a small weight problem herself, reacted hysterically, "It is completely unhealthy to lose so much in this short time. What happens if she relapses again? Also, I do not want to eat salad every day." Her reaction simply was a bursting of the balloons. In the course of her life up to now, she herself imagined her "truth." Her statement about eating salad was conjecture. The interesting thing now is that she did not ask how my girlfriend did it or what information my girlfriend followed. She simply reacted.

Another example: I once told a mother whose son attended school that I knew how understanding worked and that this method can be used by everyone. Her reaction was regarding whether this knowledge could be conveyed at all. To my astonishment, she did not even bother to find out how this method works. She was a nurse, and I believe that she was so shaped by the impossible technical language of medicine that everything else in terms of knowledge was "difficult to convey."

A third example: Thomas bought an old farmhouse in a small village. In the house, there was a steel safe that was almost two meters high and, according to the information he had, weighed about two tons. A "heavy" matter. He went ahead and started to contact various companies to get the safe out of the house to get rid of it. A farmer came along, wiggled and shook the safe, threw it down and used logs to roll it to the door. With the tractor's front loader, he hauled the safe away. The safe did not weigh two tons. It was just the information that Thomas had.

Inner voice? Some have become dependent upon it. They rely on this inner impulse without examining the actual fact. A person's warning light turns on, so he runs away and drops the matter. Usually they are the former bad experiences that warn in the present and often decide the future.

Example: If two men use the same deodorant, it does not mean that the men have the same bad character, even though the woman is "warned" of it by the smell. The woman might have been involved with someone that treated her badly and who used that same deodorant, and, as a result, she now starts to feel cautious every time she smells that deodorant. The smell of the deodorant brings forth an uneasy feeling in her every time.

Having had an "accident" with something does not mean one will experience the same accident again in the future. People and things are different. To experience something new means to let go of the past, to look at the things as they are now and not to see any comparisons with the past. The past has passed, and although it may be a good guide for the future, do not let your past dictate your future. You have to be able to experience the new in a new unit of time.

Having a relationship as a teenager is very simple. One gives the other a kiss, falls in love, and one already has a relationship. Later on, as an adult, values suddenly come into play. The human seems to get more complicated with increasing age. One uses his personal standards to assess whether he should get involved with others. This whole matter is further complicated by the experience that one has accumulated with increasing age, and this experience is used to evaluate people and situations.

In this way, the present is linked to the past. Therefore, one does not look at the now but instead "looks through one's experience" at the current situation in an attempt to try to predict the future. You assess* the person in the hope that if you were to get involved, you will not end up falling flat on your face. You do not want to have a bad experience in the future simply because you already have had bad experiences that were painful. All too often one is no longer capable of separating the past from the present. This is how the adult has become "reasonable." He operates with a mind shaped by bad experiences. See for yourself. The bad experience is always the first thing that jumps up at you, and that spreads like a wildfire within society.

Gut feeling (inner voice) is a catastrophe within the human. It is not justifiable to condemn something that one does not personally know about or that one has not experienced for himself. So be cautious of people with a strong inner voice. These individuals, who are often very sick, live in their own imagined world, do not see the present as it is and are unable to make reasonable decision. Here we go: The mind is the enemy in our own ranks. The mind with its content has the person completely under control: "The first step to personal freedom is power over one's own mind." If the human being would observe, measure and experience his surroundings, instead of thinking, this world would become a better world.

When you are thinking, ideas will come, but now it depends on you to determine which idea you give energy and which idea you will implement. Furthermore, it is worth thinking about how it is possible to do things without being thwarted by regulations, rules and "social norms of behavior."

A healthy mind in a healthy body. You can actually recognize the mental state or the illnesses of the person by the condition of his body. Also, his personal possessions and circle of friends provide information.

A healthy mind has all virtues, such as honesty, sincerity, high conception of truth, helpfulness, commitment, responsibility, high intelligence, orderliness, cleanliness, precision, and justice and is very active. This being is usually enthusiastic and highly motivated. It finds life full of pleasure and achieves its goals because there are no "counter-thoughts" to prevent it! This is the icing on the cake; however, it is very seldom found. It has all its potential, all the energy.

With increasing mental "illness," the person's abilities and virtues decrease all the more, and he becomes an inactive spectator. His energy now works against him. One can see this in a state of disorder, illnesses (a type of disorder, only at the cellular level), unreliability, and so on, simply the opposite mentioned in the above paragraph about the healthy mind. All of this happens gradually.

"Disorder indicates the degree of confusion in the person's head!"

As a rule, you will find your fellow human beings in the state of "boredom." Conversation amounts to everyday things and is not very "ingenious." The discussion participants find it somewhat difficult to adopt a different point of view. The worse off the person is, the more one encounters resistance, and good ideas are being rejected.

Your warning lights should come on when a person is often seriously ill. If the person has glandular problems (endocrine disorders) or neurological illnesses, be twice as careful. This person has the impulse to lie and cheat, to take advantage of someone and to play down serious matters. He may not be averse to sexual perversion. This person is in the process of dying slowly and will take you along on the way. It is here where you will find feigned kindness.

Remember, there are strong glandular disorders and weak ones, as well as a strong influence from the mind or less, depending on how much power the mind has or, more precisely, how many amperes flow. Furthermore, there is conditioned social behavior. Here we have the person with glandular problems who keeps meticulous order. A contradiction? Well, how long did the parents have to act on the child until it kept order, even though it was against the child's "basic attitude?" Now who do you trust more, the person whose natural behavior is orderly or the person who had to be conditioned to keep order?

In any case, illnesses are clear signs that there is something wrong with the person and that there is something not in order, and it is questionable whether the person himself has enough horsepower to prevail against a character changing impulse from his mind. At any rate, the media constantly witness misdeeds.

"Still waters run deep ..." The facade of kindness. Only our "icing on the cake" has true balance and serenity; everything else is played, and time will show you that it is so. Are you familiar with the saying, "One can smell someone good?" Another clue. The ancient Egyptians used to allow only those women who smelled good entrance to the harem.[2] They knew why. The more a person has bad smelling body odors, the more they tell you to "go away." Of course, this does not apply to garlic fans. These should be enough clues to determine whether one has found "the right one" with whom to go through life.

Another very good indicator is the ability to communicate. Think about it, when you speak with someone, the spoken word must be understood, considered and pronounced. A capable person does this very quickly, and the answer is logical because the energy flows without resistance. The more incapable a person is, the longer the answer takes, and the less logical it is because it is blocked by one's own thoughts. The more mental freedom a person has, the less he strives in accumulating matter.

A relationship should be harmonious. Harmony means unison*. One should be on the same wavelength as the partner. If the difference is too great, both will be dissatisfied, and the relationship will not last.

"He who wants to acquire health, must separate himself from the crowd of people because the masses always go against reason and always try to hide their sufferings and weaknesses" (Seneca, Roman philosopher and raw foodist*).

Only a few remain who can see through their eyes, the rest peek through the mind and do not see the truth.

Emotion

What is emotion? Little seems to be recognizable through the word itself. Emotion = Movement. The fact is that the body is moved by emotion, or the person himself is moved by emotion. Death is not an emotion. One could inject all kinds of hormones, drugs or medication into a dead body, and there is no more emotion!

Take a small child who is still emotionally impartial in regard to social patterns. Let us assume that the child wants a piece of chocolate. He enthusiastically goes to his parents to have a piece of chocolate. He is rejected. The initial enthusiasm decreases, and the child becomes a little more reserved. The next request is rejected again. Now the interest levels off, and the child gets angry, screams or starts to cry. If the parents remain tough, the child will no longer want any chocolate out of sheer spite or resignation (apathy), at least in this current emotional state.

There is an emotional band area that the person lives through every day: Successes or good news raise the emotional level, whereby losses, defeats and bad news lower it. Over time, the person's general emotional level drops due to mistakes, bad experiences or just one blow of fate, and he seems to be stuck in the lower area. In any case, adults are at a different emotional level than children. Face it, who can show more enthusiasm for something than a child?

A scale of emotions.[2] The following is a brief presentation of the emotional scale without listing the subtleties: enthusiasm, strong interest, conservatism*, boredom, antagonism, anger, grief, apathy* and death. Every emotional level has its own peculiarities, like thinking, behaving, the state of the body, and so on. Remember, the organism is flooded with adrenaline* when one is angry to activate physical energy.

In fact, an entire section of study of over several thousand pages on this subject is presented in the books of L. Ron Hubbard. At this point, I do not wish to address specialized knowledge to illuminate emotion scientifically. It is enough to observe oneself and to realize that there is emotion. Emotions are measurable values; they are wavelengths. One can tell from the other person's voice if he is enthusiastic, bored or angry. On closer inspection, one has to assume that the vocal cords have to be set in an exact movement. So, there is an energy impulse on the vocal cords that causes the movement, as well as the heart rate.

Unfortunately, conventional* science is not advanced enough to present a plausible* theory since there is very little functional knowledge of electrical energy. The vocal cords are weakly controlled electrically; it is an impulse*. If electrical energy were "free conducting electrons*" or photons*, a precise control would not be possible. It is a direct control, like the forward or backward movement of a lever. If this were not the case, one would not have precise control! In this way, the entire neural system is controlled, including the glands.

In medicine, one hears that hormones cause feelings, but it is exactly the other way around. The glands must first receive the energy impulse before they release hormones. The person must first become angry before the body adapts to the "wavelength of anger." If one were to designate the person as a function and the body as a structure, then the function would be superior to the structure, for example, mind over matter. "Aha" thinks the medical professional, "What happens in the case of an injury? First there is the external impulse that activates the body's defense measures! This means that the structure affects the function." Oh well, as I said, a dead body does nothing more, even if one amputates its leg. In the event of an injury, the injured area "reports" the injury with an impulse, considering that the body is an organized arrangement of cells in which every single cell* lives for itself. This impulse is evaluated, and so another impulse from the control center (the person, not the brain) is sent to initiate countermeasures.

Enough theory! I mean, the human wants a measured value and an explanation of why things are. He does not like to simply believe and needs a solid reference.

What is it really about? Well, the human educates his peers not to live out their emotions. For example: "A native American knows no pain." "Boys don't cry." "He who is angry is not in control of himself!"

Emotions are a "catalyst"* for the experiences of this world. If someone is angry, he should be angry; if someone is sad, he should cry! He will cry or be angry until the energy impulse is completely exhausted. Only by living out an emotion will he move to the next higher emotional level right up to cheerful serenity, which is above enthusiasm. If the emotion is not lived out, the energy impulse is not exhausted and will continue to affect the body. There you have it: *Mens sana in corpore sano**! (A sound mind in a sound body.)

The physical state is a direct indicator of the emotional state. People in an emotional state of fear are often sick, have glandular problems and possess a gloomy outlook on life. A lot of money is spent on social security. The environment is messy, like the mind. There is a tendency towards irresponsibility, such that one is rather willing to accept things instead of doing something. It should be noted here that upbringing is an influencing factor. Upbringing actually is superordinate pressure. The parents work on their children until they are "brought up," just like the government with citizens. If the pressure was big enough and long enough, this behavior pattern is adopted contrary to the "natural orientation."

The emotion fear has a very specific function; one becomes hypersensitive and the senses sharpen. The concentration remains fixed with the perceptions. The external order plays little or no role because "danger" is imminent. Remember, the person is afraid! Hands and feet become damp to increase the grip on the subsurface, useful for a better escape, be it now up a tree or out of the danger zone entirely. To detect if a person is in an "anxious state," there may be body odors due to perspiration. It is not to be expected that this person thinks rationally because he is afraid.

The environment actually is the determining factor in how any organism reacts towards the situation. With anger, strengths are activated that one "normally" does not have; one tends to attack or defend oneself hard.

In turn, boredom relaxes the entire physical system, the attention being scattered, whereas the attention is fixed again with "interest," but this time on a rational level to evaluate information or a situation. Interest is in the upper band area. Roughly, one could put the emotional levels in relation to free mental energy. This means that the lower the level, the less mental ability and virtue, the higher, the more responsible, more capable ability to recognize the world in its entirety, including the ability to distinguish the individual parts and to act accordingly. Sitting there in untouchable serenity and doing nothing that some have considered sacred is probably unrelated to mental health!

The reason for the emotions of the organism may lay completely in the evolution based on the time of "teeth and claws" when it was about defending the organism against attacking carnivores. Mind you, I am talking about the organism because animals have emotions, as do plants. It is "life" that expresses the emotion with the intention of protecting the organism or reacting correctly emotionally in the respective situation. Real reason can only be expected in the presence of balance and serenity, not under pressure!

Now we are out of the "teeth and claws" stage, but the same emotions are still effective. The above is only a basic insight into how life affects the organism through emotion, which means that the human can be understood as a living being when he expresses emotion and acts and decides on the basis of it. To emphasize it again in conclusion: There is nothing wrong with emotions; they are part of life. Experience them!

Love

Oh, yes, love, I almost forgot. Well, what is that anyway? I do not believe that there is anything that seems more important to the human being. You love the things you want to have the most. One would do almost anything to get what one loves the most. It is a feeling, a sensation that seems to lift you to a higher plane - level of happiness, hope and soulfulness - Heaven on Earth.

And yet this feeling arises from yourself. It is just that you are wrongly assigning the cause by believing that you are given this feeling by something or someone else. The sensation of love is not an earthly thing. It is not made of matter nor is it a thing of God because He does not give you the sensation. It is something that has to do with yourself.

However, love is the most interpreted, misused and misunderstood word. Actually, the word loving, by origin, means making something pleasant for someone. Now see for yourself because it is a simple matter to love the pleasant aspects of life. There are basically three types (LRH):

1. The purely sexual impulse: This is "love at first sight." It can be a very strong feeling. But unfortunately, this feeling is no guarantee for a lasting relationship. By not really being on a similar wavelength, the initial strong affection eventually will turn into the opposite. This can go on for years with one

getting a bit more unhappy every day.

2. Compulsive love: One has a craving for a partner, although one is mistreated and betrayed by him. This feeling is an indication that a thought has power over the person. The thought commands, and the person obeys.

3. Real affection: This can only be achieved if the chemistry is right. The top maxim* for maintaining harmony is good communication. One can truly talk about anything and is understood. However, to do this, two beings must be in a good state. Sadly, the divorce rate of today's society shows that this is not the case.

Hence, one really should be careful not to be fooled by this feeling. Do not think with your genitals, but instead think about how you can live life with your partner without getting burned. Remember, love takes freedom. Some individuals become unhappy in a relationship because they have given up too much of their free time. Nevertheless, one can have a happy relationship and still cultivate other interests. First, one has to come to terms with oneself, divide his time and, for once, let the relationship be a relationship – just switch off from it.

Speaking of the definition of love, L. Ron Hubbard said, it is "the desire to occupy the same space as the other." This would be the maximum degree of love, but even here there is a gradient scale. The opposite of that would be hatred, and when you truly hate someone, you will avoid or even fight him. Thus, love and hate have a lot to do with space.

There still is an old word that is related to this subject: affinity*. Affinity could be described as inclination. It is exactly what holds a relationship together. The opposite of that would be disinclination. By disinclining from someone, one does not have a good relationship. Affection has a lot to do with commonness. By having something in common with someone, one is inclined to him. When there is no one with whom one has something in common, one is lonely. Having coinciding* interests leads to common ground; disagreement and argument leads to loneliness. The only thing that holds this world and this universe together is affinity – also at the molecular level.

Attractiveness and Character

In terms of character, I believe the above explanation is more than adequate. The second dynamic is ultimately about preserving the race – in purely biological terms.

How does that beautiful saying go, "One also eats with one's eyes." So, keep yourself attractive. Attractive means to attract, which brings us back to the topics of inclination and disinclination. One feels like doing something when one likes it and when it gives one pleasure.

Being delectable has something to do with taking care of one's body. My former girlfriend Kerstin is a brilliant example. Dissatisfied in the last relationship, she put on a few extra pounds, 103 kilograms (227 pounds) to be exact. All previous "diets" had been unsuccessful, and she also had a loss in the quality of life because she could not really eat her fill and could not eat what she liked. Consequently, I suggested that she read *Fit for Life*[3] because, as some of you may already know, it is important to be informed before doing anything. More than a "diet" book, this book conveys an attitude towards life, and Kerstin is still totally fascinated with it. She often cooks with friends and can eat as much as she desires. Her weight now? She went from 103 kilograms in 2000 to 57 kilograms (125 pounds) in 2003 – all a matter of "know how!" She is also very proud of herself and rightly so. She told me that the opposite gender is now also turning its head towards her - no wonder! ☺

All too often, beauty is associated with women, but men can be attractive as well. One just has to do something for oneself. As already mentioned, the problem starts in the head, and it is noticeable on the body!

The value of beauty as a subject actually requires independent work to sufficiently exhaust it. Beauty and aesthetics seem to be of the greatest value for the human being. Viewed from the effect side*, it could also be described as pleasing. The matter is a very simple one. One surrounds oneself with the things that one likes and disposes of them when one no longer likes them.

The human first tries to please himself. He scrutinizes himself in front of the mirror to somehow look good. See for yourself. Women put on make-up, choose special clothing and accessories (jewelry, scarfs, and so on) and select stylish shoes. Guys almost do the same, except that with them, it should be "cool," to use a word from today's jargon*.

Character*? The person insists on being accepted as he or she is? Hmm, maybe that should be reconsidered. What happens if the other person does not like it at all?

Remember, beauty is that something with which one can be caught most easily because one wants to have it! At second glance, one will recognize the background: admiration. Beauty and admiration go hand in hand. When one finds things beautiful, one admires them; thus admiration has the highest power. Admiration has a very wide range; one can be admired for many things, be it beauty, performance in sport or character. One loves the things that one admires.

A Few Words About "Life"

Life consists of eight driving forces or dynamics (LRH):

The first dynamic is you, yourself, with your very personal goals and intentions. This would be the self-momentum.

The second dynamic is reproduction. This includes the opposite gender and the raising of children.

The third dynamic is the group dynamic. This would be your place of work, your football club or a locality or nation that one can describe as a group. You live with and through a group.

The fourth dynamic is humanity. You belong in this grouping as well, and you would defend humanity in an attack by aliens.

The fifth dynamic would be subordinate living beings, as well as animals and plants. This is another part of this world, and you live with them and through them.

The sixth dynamic is the matter dynamic. This is the ground you stand on, the house you live in and the car that you drive.

The seventh dynamic is you as a spiritual being, the part that organizes and keeps everything together.

The eighth dynamic is God or Infinity*.

Every human being has all of these driving forces. He only has more preferences for one or the other. However, if one of those dynamics were to be completely removed, the human, as such, would perish. This is precisely why one should ensure that each of these dynamics is preserved, and this can be achieved by investing time and tending to the matter. In other words, this means not just working all the time or hanging out with one's boy or girlfriend!

By limiting oneself to just one or two dynamics, the greater part of life is lost. Every dynamic has a right to exist. To give up a dynamic means to give up on oneself.

Life on the dynamics has four essential points:

1. Knowledge
2. Trust

3. Winning

4. To be free from

So, let us put this into practice. Of course, you will be able to trust only to the extent that you know something about a matter. Winning means that if you say "yes" to something, you also mean "yes," and if you say "no," you also mean "no." You have to rely on and believe in yourself and not let yourself be fooled.

To be free from means that you can separate yourself from the part that makes up a dynamic. For example: Realizing that your current job will harm others and that you might end up in jail, you have to break away from this job. Hence, you will be free from it. Of course, you also will be able to do something else.

Separate yourself from the things that do more harm than good to you!

The same goes for a relationship. It applies to all dynamics. The area of knowledge that deals with these driving forces is called ethics. Ethics has its own laws and demonstrates how a happy existence is possible.

Exchange Factors

There are four exchange factors in number (LRH):

1. **Taking without giving.** This is what a thief or criminal would do.
2. **Taking a lot and giving a little.** Not quite as criminal but unfair. This is what governments or big industries do.
3. **Fair exchange.** One takes as much as one gives. This is found among good craftsmen.
4. **Giving a little more than taking.** This includes a good product, delivered quickly with friendly service. One orients oneself to the wishes of the customer, whereby the extras are also included in the price. One can turn a blind eye to minor things. The rise or fall depends on the exchange factors. In the end, you decide whether you can live with number four, like the maggot in the Speck*, or whether you slowly perish with number two. The exchange factors are used in every area of human activity: in love, in society, in politics, at the doctor, or even when writing a letter.

The Definition of Reason

1. Doing or refraining from actions that will bring you and your symbionts* more advantages than disadvantages, even in the future.

2. "Reason is the leading of an organism along the eight dynamics towards pleasure." (LRH)

The organism is the body that you have grabbed and lead through space and time. This would be the definition of life - without you there is no life! Life is fun when one is motivated. One is motivated when one has fun or works towards it.

You are a friend to this world and your fellow human beings when you are reasonable.

If one only has suppression, pain and loss, one would not be motivated. One would be listless and would have no joy in life. By the way, suppression causes illness. A good being loses his worth in a suppressive environment.

So, be reasonable and ensure that you have fun in life! But consider: The sword of ethics hovers over all existence. Ethics are possessed and owned by the individual. By violating them, there is a judge who knows no mercy - you yourself. Remember, accidents and mishaps do not happen in vain! **Additionally, when your ethic fails, the law comes into play.**

Responsibility
Ensuring Things Go Well

To ensure means doing something effectively and not just talking about it! In the word responsibility is the word *response*. Well, one can only respond to something by knowing something about it! Thus, there is a direct relationship between knowledge and responsibility. By having knowledge about a matter or a thing, one can deal with it and can control it.

Let us take a car as an example. A car is known to consume oil. It is also known that the engine breaks down without oil. So, one could say that the operator of this car is responsible for the engine oil level.

This is a simple example of how the operator of a thing is responsible for something. To the extent that he is responsible, he should also be liable, that is, if he causes harm, he should make amends for it.

Responsibility arises from knowing; it is something that one has. One can only bear this responsibility by knowing. Telling someone to be responsible (liable) for this can only work if the person is educated about it.

Of course, it is puzzling to appoint someone as the Minister of Defense who has not previously served in an appropriate position in an army for some period of time or to appoint a Minister of Transport who did not even work as a driving instructor for a few years. These guys do not know their way around, and they can be misled by their "consultants." Incompetent.

This is similar to a teacher. How can he "educate" without the basic knowledge about the mind and understanding.

Incidentally, everyone who takes over a post should receive a written job description with all of the details that also includes all of the people that are necessary to carry out the work. This job description, of course, should be written by the person who previously held the post.

An employee will be able to work exactly only to the extent that he has learned and practiced every activity. It is of no use to say, "Plaster this wall!" It is better to demonstrate and to explain **how** the work can be done. Guiding principle: **"Something takes too long; something goes terribly wrong."**

In a civilization with complicated and expensive technology, mistakes can have fatal consequences, be it in an activity or in training. When everyone bears his responsibility or passes on things that extend into another area of responsibility, then there can be a togetherness and a system can work.

To stand there and to announce with great pride and with one's head held high, "I take full responsibility!", only to throw in the towel by giving up the post is not taking responsibility but deserting*one's post, like the authorities usually practice. These individuals probably should be held accountable, including their private assets to see to it that they make up for the mess that they have caused, while receiving a million-dollar compensation for their "services." Where did we ever end up?! Offer the other cheek, also?

In fact, it is so that "your sins are forgiven" brings forth a decadent* society. One should act in repairing the damage that one has caused. Furthermore, it has been shown that "sins" as represented in the Catholic Church do not have much in common with right and wrong. What has proven itself in mental processes is that if one does bad things, bad things will befall one. By taking responsibility and implementing it, one can determine one's fate and counteract bad karma*.

Responsibility (a full definition): Recognizing a grievance and bringing forth a constructive idea in regard to reason*. The decision to remedy the grievance and to implement the idea includes one fully accepting the consequences of one's original action and working on the grievance until a satisfactory conclusion has been reached.

This applies not only if one makes a mistake but also in the performance of any activity or, rather, the handling of materials. Routine work is as much a responsibility as the reason for the person performing this work.

Well, how about if each of us took the full definition of responsibility as a principle for life? What kind of world would we have then?

Responsibility in a 2D? One should have some understanding about humans, why he thinks the way he thinks and why he acts the way he acts. One knows a lot about a healthy relation, if the goals and intentions of the partner are known, which he tries to achieve with and by a relationship. If one can get one's goals and intentions in line with the one's of the partner, one just needs to work on them.

Happiness:

"The overcoming of not unknown obstacles towards a known goal" (LRH). Think about what it was like when the examiner told you that you had passed the driving exam. You were happy! You can set your own goals and achieve them. It is your action, your doing. It is how you determine your tomorrow, your future, no more and no less!

Your future? It is within you; it is in what you have planned for tomorrow and what you want to achieve. When you have achieved all of your goals, then you no longer have a future; therefore, set new goals for yourself that you want to achieve! People who died soon after they retired died for exactly that reason: There was no more task, and there was nothing left that they could achieve! Also, keep in mind that no one will bring you a bucket full of happiness; you have to work on it yourself.

Happiness and Freedom?

Happiness begins with the strive to have something. Then when one has it, the sensations are twofold: to be glad to have it and the worry of losing it, which adds a somewhat bitter taste to the actual happiness. Ultimately, things are lost, and one is unhappy.

So, what do we learn from it? Is it desirable to renounce everything in order not to experience loss in life? To sit down like a yogi* under a tree, to meditate and to hold up an arm* until it dies? To let life pass by completely?

Life means to be there for life, to do decent work so that life can live! One has no other choice but to experience the events in life, every happiness and every pain.

The real ability lies in the ability to have freedom itself. Freedom means that one does **not** have to have that something that makes one happy because to have to have it and to not get it is infinite* suffering. It is the greed that arises from spiritual poverty to have nothing else. There is nothing wrong with having something, but there is a lot wrong with being "dependent" on something and to do everything possible to keep it!

Happiness lies in being able to create new things over and over again, to be able to experience something new and to have the ability to let go of the old. It is a mental process, a work with thoughts. Your happiness and your freedom lie in the thoughts themselves.

Unhappiness

Has the person become unhappy? Has his laughter completely ceased? Well, that is because he had to accept too many losses and rejections, and he was denied experiencing things. So, what could be done to have a world full of happy people? Well, find out what makes the human happy and give him the opportunity to achieve it! Have you not noticed that every time you make someone happy, you get a little bit of that feeling of happiness?

The Human's Will is His Kingdom of Heaven

What is the will of the human being? What is it made of? The body alone results in a certain need. It should be maintained at a moderate temperature, fed and protected from the forces of nature. A sexual impulse should also ensure that the species itself is preserved.

Well, that is actually all there is to say! Everyone probably has noticed that it is not so easy after all. There is something that feels the temperature, judges the taste of the food, wants to dress nicely and is very picky about the choice of a partner. It is the person himself who decides what he wants. But on what basis does he decide? He decides between the things he knows about and what he thinks will bring him joy and no harm.

Do not believe that the terms joy and harm are chosen carelessly, no matter how awkward they may sound. Just take a look at your surrounding area. Every article fulfills a task - the ballpoint pen, the sheet of paper, the chair, the bed and your partner in life with whom you share the time. All of these things are friends to you because they serve you. Now imagine that these things would do exactly the opposite of what you expected them to do - catastrophe! Consequently, you can make the decision based on joy and harm!

By getting something or doing something now, you will be extra careful so that it is safe, or you will somehow try to make it safe! What I mean by that is that you want to have your money when you have worked for it. You want your shoes to last and feel comfortable when walking in them. The hotel for your vacation should keep the promises in its brochure and not be a construction site! You want security, security to the extent that you will be able to live out your ideas, your ideas being that something from which your will results!

Recently I was talking to my female dentist. She told me that people were coming to her in rows and wanted to have their amalgam fillings* removed from their teeth. Thereupon my female dentist said, "I let my patients decide freely!" "Well," I said to her, "based on what information?!"

In fact, science is not necessarily scientific because someone is constantly inventing a theory that nobody understands any more. A scientist lets out a bad word, brings forth a "plausible theory" about it, and everyone starts to panic. Why? Mass medium television! What exactly do you see in this box? Danger, a theory to protect yourself and to give you security, and of course the product for it! Opinion making and manipulation!

And do not believe for a second that what you get out of this box will not affect you in some way. Should you get into a situation similar to that shown on television, you will fall back on this information that has been given to you, unless you are better off and have broadened your mental horizon in this regard! For example, my mother was sitting in front of the television and watched a car overturn at a rally*. "Funny," she said, "the car does not explode at all!" Well, in Hollywood movies, they do that constantly. However, gasoline is not an explosive; it burns, but it does not explode! For this reason, the first responder* at the scene of the accident still has some time to get the injured person out of the car, even when it is on fire, unless the first responder has too much Hollywood on his mind!

Who does not allow a few extra dollars to be pulled out of their pockets for security reasons? No matter how invented and inaccessible the security may be.

The idea that results in the will? Everyone is probably familiar with hypochondria: the patient who imagines his illness. In fact, one probably first "had enough" before one has a cold. The stress at work has become too great or the relationship has gone completely off the rails. One wants some distance, a timeout and actually maneuvers himself offside - and one becomes ill.

Study of medicine? Illnesses are described in detail, and one gets a very precise idea of what is happening. The student worries about all that he might have or even develops the exact phenomena as described! However, one thing has completely faded into the background. The person is not his body!

"The thoughts are free." I believe that they have long been put into chains, been classified and are subject to censorship*!

Remember: If you want to make someone happy with a gift, find out what they want because, no matter what you think, the recipient may think very differently! Obtruding* one's will on another? How would you feel if someone were to do that to you? What could be nicer then living in one's own heavenly kingdom? The only question is, "With whom do I share it, and how can my heavenly kingdom be that of the other?"

Loyalty, Fidelity and Happiness

Well, this topic seems important enough to me to write something about it. However, I have the idea that I will be embarking on very treacherous* terrain here. Among other things, this topic has a lot to do with humanity instead of reason, in other words, with objective clear thinking. Loyalty is often equated with fidelity*, even though the word loyalty has been taken by the government. Why? Loyalty comes from legal, which could also be called "legally." In this sense, the definition is articulated: Faithful to the law or loyal to an employer.

In turn, fidelity is held in high regard as a human virtue – a trait*. One could define fidelity with the negative, one does not cheat, or the positive, to continue to pursue a common goal and keep mutual promises. Regarding virtue, it could be said that one is good for something. So, is the human good for fidelity? As discussed in previous texts, one definition of reason is the pursuit of pleasure. So, now try to reconcile fidelity with reason!? A nice headache!

It is called so beautifully: One wants the other to be loyal, which applies in every relationship, be it in an interpersonal relationship between the sexes or in the relationship between the individual and the employer, association or country.

Whom or what is one actually loyal to? The human often uses the words fidelity and loyalty only to exploit* the human for personal gain and to make him feel guilty – nothing there!

It is neither the partner, the employer nor the country to which you are loyal! In the following example, you will recognize that it is goals and intentions to which one is loyal, not persons or institutions, the workplace and the government being counted as institutions.

The first definition of reason has been discussed already; however, I will bring it to mind again: "The carrying out and/or the omitting of actions, which will also bring more advantages than disadvantages for you and your symbionts in the future." So, starting from this point, you are first of all being true to your basic intention, which would be to survive as an individual. If you were a hero, you would sacrifice your life in an emergency if it could be seen that by doing this, you could save your family, your country and your fellow human beings. Thus, the definition of reason is still valid; one life stands for the fate of maybe 1000 lives.

In this sense, you also would be loyal to a party or the government if it continues to pursue positive goals for the citizen, unless you see only the personal benefit, which sooner or later will break your neck! It would be sensible to be loyal to a government if it governed for the citizen and not advocated for the position and livelihood of various politicians or officials. If it is not for the citizen, why should the citizen be loyal to it? In this sense, the individual citizen also should consider for whom he is fighting the war!

Through your work for your employer, who is your bread and butter, the first basis for existence is fulfilled; therefore, you remain loyal to him as long as he contributes with money or goods to your survival. However, this is bought loyalty, as you will likely change employers in the hope for advancement.

Your second basic intention is to be happy; this is the following thing to which you are faithful after survival! I believe that if you were extremely unhappy in your current job, you would change it, even if you would earn less in another position. Happiness could be described as the human's greatest good. It is what the human strives for the most. Happiness is a state of mind. The opposite of happy would be unhappy.

An unhappy human being is demotivated, and he has a hard time pulling himself together to be active. He and his surroundings suffer from negligence; his attention to things is weak; he is indifferent; his susceptibility to accidents is high; and, he is susceptible to illnesses. An unhappy human being can be a danger to his environment; one could say that he is a heavy ballast.

Actually, in this regard, there should be laws that will help unhappy human beings be happy. After all, the human has a right to happiness; however, this is not anchored as a separate section in human rights. A truly happy human wants to live! Just as he wants to live, he is aware that the things he needs to live must be in good condition in order to be used in life. In fact, he will not be tolerant toward things, himself, his family, his work, the government, his country or the world. Only someone who is truly happy will be fully responsible for things, and by that I mean, it is not indifferent to him!

Now in regard to the interpersonal area. Fraud is a breach of trust. Up to that point, fraud is an unfair matter because the boundaries have not been clarified beforehand. Being unfaithful means having a sexual relationship with someone else, either because one is not happy in a relationship in this sense or because one has no control over one's libido (impulse to reproduce). If this is the case, one should avoid this person or, if one belongs to this group of people, one should point this out to the future partner and clarify boundaries.

I believe that the individual no longer likes to have sex with his partner when he knows that he or she is maintaining other sexual relationships. Regarding this point, it is also very sensible and a matter of self-protection because there are still many sexually transmitted diseases (STDs*) ☹. However, some biologists hold that polygamy* (sex with multiple people) would be more conducive to the preservation of the human species. However, one should consider this very carefully, as frequent changes in sexual partners can also spread a deadly virus.

When I remember my first relationship, I find that there was insufficient communication to disclose personal desires to make it possible to set common goals and objectives. At the beginning of a relationship, it may be only an affair, but in the long term, one should state exactly what one desires with and through a relationship.

As mentioned above, the second basic intention is happiness. One should actually promise one's partner this, by saying, "I want to make you happy." Of course, you have to find out what makes your partner happy. In this sense, the mutual goals and intentions have to be coordinated. This often includes compromises, and it also should be ensured that everyone is assured personal freedom. Consider: Even decisions take time.

This is the only guarantee for a relationship in which one is working towards mutual happiness. Should one ever get truly unhappy in a relationship, then one will decide against that relationship!

In a long-term relationship, one is often only satisfied. By that I mean, one can be happy and satisfied or just satisfied. It is up to oneself to maintain this state until the end of one's life. One should be true to one's own happiness and, in a relationship, ensure that the other one is happy as well. Should one become unhappy, one should find out why, clear the boundaries and again work toward being happy, if there is a need to be with another partner.

But how can you be happy in this world? You delight in something, and it is taken from you, be it your hard-earned money through high taxes, another decides against you, or a great misfortune comes your way. But as long as there still is a spark of life in you, you can do something. You can bring things to life!

Faithfulness does not have to be something to hold onto obsessively, only to be unhappy with it and to waste one's life!

P.S. When making a promise, only promise what you really want and what you can keep. Do not exceed your area of competence*!

Maintain the same attitude with your surrounding and pass this on for reading. (Dedicated to Kerry.)

Do You Know Who Your Friends Are?

Let us take the word *friend*. What is included in this word? Friend, friendly. Hence, something that gives you pleasure. A friend is someone who brings you joy. Consequently, there are friends, big and small. Giving joy has a lot to do with how much another is beneficial for your existence. You are happy when someone helps you out of a jam or with the smaller things in life that tell you that you are not alone when someone else gives you a few minutes and is kind and polite to you. To feel joy in being and to enjoy life are things a friend can give you, making him deserving of the name friend.

So how does one classify a friend, or how does one know what a friend is and what a friend is not? I had asked myself this question long ago. As a child, someone was a friend when one liked him well. This being "well-liked" resulted from pursuing common interests. One thought the same or similar because one was probably the same age and underwent the same training. One did not tease the other because they were about equal and trusted one another, even at a young age. All in all, this interpersonal relationship worked because a lot was the same or similar, and the differences were not that great.

But childhood friendships can end due to great differences and breaks in trust. Here, it is interesting to note that this is also the reason why adult friendships divide or cannot exist. A friend is someone who has the same intentions, and a foe* is just the opposite. He has intentions that are directed against your intentions; thus, he cherishes different thoughts. If everyone were to think the same thought or to coordinate with one another, then everyone could be a friend to everyone.

A friend is someone who is there for you in times of need and who helps you to survive. It is not the drinking buddy or anyone you like well for any reason. These people merely serve for your entertainment and are colleagues or comrades. Actual friends are the baker who gives you your bread, the craftsmen who build your house for you, the repair shop owner who repairs your car, and all that for a fair price. Ensure that your friends also can be there for you later.

"Help is help as long as one gets something in return; otherwise, it is a fraud or a crime." Therefore, if you do something for your buddy, he owes you something, if not right away, then later. Remember: One hand washes the other; whoever takes, also has to give.

Friendship has a big separation point: help. Breaches of trust may be detrimental; however, real help results in gratitude! I believe that if someone has really been helped, he or she will gladly help the one who has helped.

All too often one hears of a "help-syndrome." A syndrome is a condition characterized by a set of associated symptoms related to collapse in a certain clinical picture – as if help had something to do with illness. Without help, nothing would work on this planet. None of us would have made it to adulthood without being helped! Help makes a difference; it shows the value of a person. A friend will not let one down.

So, what essentially constitutes a real friendship? Basis: Associate with one another in an appropriate tone (actually, I should write politely and kindly, which would be desirable) and take the other as he or she is. Mmm, occasionally! Two human beings, two ideas - one has to meet somewhere.

One wants:
- Honesty and sincerity and not to be exploited.
- The other to be there when one needs him or her.
- Confidential matters treated confidentially.
- One to respect the other as an individual and give him or her free space.
- The other to help one when one is facing difficulty.
- Someone who can take care of his own area and environment and who likes to give advice.

- Someone who will not let one down.
- Someone who does not betray another.
- Someone that one can trust.
- Someone with whom one can laugh.
- Someone with whom one can "steal horses."
- Someone to whom one can tell everything.
- Someone who stands behind one.
- Someone whom one can help and who accepts help.
- Someone who at times leaves one be.
- Someone who still knows a person, even if they have not seen one another for a long time.
- Someone who can forgive another.
- Someone who gives one a piece of his or her mind or shares an honest opinion.
- Someone with whom one can share something, such that he or she takes care of it and gives it back safely – and not after months!
- Someone, who even after a long friendship, knows the difference between mine, yours and together, depending on how it was acquired.
- Someone who holds me back when I am about to do something stupid.
- Someone with whom one can also go other ways.
- Someone who also tolerates and accepts other friends.
- Someone who keeps his or her moods and whims to himself.
- Someone who is capable of criticism and who works on himself.
- Someone who supports and motivates a person, instead of putting him down.
- Someone who will maintain my original intention when I get fickle*.
- Someone who acknowledges logic and who seeks possibilities instead of simply saying, "No."
- Someone who does not have to be in the right.
- Someone to whom one listens and understands.

Give it some thought. Maybe there are a few more things that make a real friendship for you.

Trust the other blindly? Do not do it! Verify things yourself to be sure that any contracts are understood or that the work is done correctly or that materials are flawless.

Not doing this yourself means making a pact with uncertainty. It follows that because you are not completely knowledgeable and because things can happen unexpectedly with which you do not agree, you will blame the other. So, because you do not see the need for certainty and because you do not take responsibility for the things you have gotten yourself into, it is easy to blame the person who recommended, sold or repaired the item for you. Simply accusing and assigning blame to the other completely ruins the mutual relationship!

For this reason, check contracts, work, materials, service that was rendered and clarify the matters with which you do not agree right away because later on there will only be a lot of hassle! Prevent it for the sake of yourself and your fellow human beings!

To be for the other? To give him or her the last of your money? Do **not** do it! When you have enough money, you can give it freely, but always consider your livelihood, because when you have given everything, you end up in the "devil's kitchen." But remember, in this society, you are only as stable as your ability to help yourself, and this helping yourself is too often based on only one thing: money! Therefore, be responsible and self-sufficient because asking the other for help can get him into trouble, too.

As already indicated in the previous articles: Use this document and pass it on to your fellow human beings. And if you have a real friend, make him aware of the various points if he has violated them or does not properly pay attention to them. A real friendship is more valuable than money; therefore, work on it to preserve it.

Everything can be solved with direct and factual communication. For this reason, keep your emotions under control and remember that you also have made mistakes!

Friendships exist mainly because there are many likenesses and similarities or because a game is played in which there is a common goal. Special associations are formed in the fight against a common opponent.

A difficult question is: What is worth more, a love affair or a real friendship? In a friendship, one can tell one another more or do things without hurting the other emotionally, which guarantees a longer existence. On the other hand, love affairs are very fragile matters because the average person has enough problems with him or herself, and, by adding a life partner, it becomes all the more difficult. Nevertheless, the explanations of what really makes a real friendship also apply here. Read the second dynamic code.

Personally, I would not risk a real friendship because of a love affair. You are married? How high is the divorce rate, and who is still there afterwards? Two more sentences: **"Show me your friends, and I will tell you who you are. You will recognize them by their actions"** (LRH).

We have to get along with the human beings who are here ... there are no others. We are all sitting in the same boat called planet Earth. It should be noted here that the time may come when some will relocate and maybe get to know other worlds and beings; thus, the boat gets all the bigger.

Since this boat is quite large, one will not meet one or the other in the course of a lifetime, and one easily can avoid another. However, one should always be aware of one thing and that is to always avoid an idea, probably even one's own. Problems only arise from fixed ideas* and the inability to look closely at them and change them. What I mean is: One wants to be in the right, or, perhaps more correctly, one has to be right.

Living together requires mutual acceptance and tolerance. The belief of one does not necessarily have to be that of the other. However, one should be able to accept the things around one and realize that they exist no matter from where they ultimately come.

As for the crew on the boat, we do not control this planet, but it has to work somehow, and often there are almost mysterious ways of how to meet one or the other again. In this sense, one should be friendly towards one's contemporaries and treat them accordingly and also part in peace. One never knows in what hardship one might meet someone.

As mentioned in "Orientation," **Why should I have you as an enemy when I can have you as a friend!** Bear in mind: One does not have to be a friend to everyone – treat an idiot as befits an idiot!

PS: It is up to oneself with whom one chooses to have real friendships.

The Problem Begins in the Head
Definition of problem: intention, counter intention (LRH).

Example: You are sitting in the car with the intention of starting the engine. It does not work. Somewhere there is a "counter intention." Hence, you have a problem!

You now have the following options:
1. Increase your intention.
2. Remove the counter intention.

Application:

1. You try again and again.
2. You check the starter, the battery, the cable, and so on, and remove the source of the error. If you are unable to do it, then the repair shop will.

Every problem consists of intention and counter intention, even in your own head, as described at the beginning of this chapter. The handling is always the same, even in the interpersonal area.

A problem arises like a squeaking noise, a strange smell, and somehow things get difficult and deviate from a normal course. Find the real cause and react appropriately in time before problems get big and too expensive. Follow guidelines so that you do not get into such a mess again!

What about a problem that just does not want to go away? It is the lie that lets things exist! For example, your car's engine is not running properly, and you drive it to the repair shop. There you are told that the control unit is defective and must be replaced. Once repaired, you find that the engine is still not running properly – so the defective control unit was a lie, since the problem still exists. Following this, the software for the control unit is updated, but the problem still exists. Later on, it turns out that the skilled worker is not a trained mechanic, but a butcher, and the customer accidentally had filled up with diesel instead of gasoline. Thus, the truth was a bogus mechanic and wrong fuel, and handling those circumstances solved the problem.

Problems just do not go away. Well, where are all the lies?

Anatomy* of a Problem

Well, what is a problem, and when does one have a problem? One always has a problem with something, be it with a thing, a condition, a person, a situation or oneself.

One has a problem when one gets involved with something. A problem exists when one has agreed that it exists.

I mean, look, you first have to get involved with something before you have a problem with it. And on closer inspection, you find that there is always a problem with yourself. You have the idea of how it should be, but the reality is different; therefore, you have a problem. Reality is always the product of someone else's idea, which brings us to intention and counter intention. Intention simply means the attempt of carrying out an idea.

Let us say that you had a problem with mathematics. So, you got involved with mathematics. The problem revealed is that you did not understand the rules upon which mathematics is based; therefore, you did not achieve the results that you actually should have achieved. That is because the rules of mathematics are someone else's ideas. So, by understanding and agreeing with these rules, you can deliver the corresponding results. Now, you no longer have a problem because you basically agreed to this thing called mathematics.

Unfortunately, you are more or less forced to agree and get involved with various things. If you do not master some part of mathematics, you will not receive a secondary school certificate or an apprenticeship, and, without an apprenticeship, you will be unable to get a job to earn a living. Thus, problems are created for you.

But apart from that, there is another way. An old friend of mine, who is a self-employed entrepreneur in the plastering trade, has neither learned the profession nor completed his master craftsman diploma, and I do not know whether he actually has a secondary school certificate. However, it does not matter. Well, he started as an assistant and was clever enough to understand the trade in order to practice it. He simply hired a master plasterer and instantly became the boss of the company. From my previous findings so far, I have to say, thank God he left school early because doing so saved his mind, as education tends to mess up the mind of the individual with strange ideas.

In any case, he mastered the basic mathematical and the area and percentage calculations, exactly what is needed in the trade. Because he still had a clear mind and could add one plus one together, he was able to run a company successfully, which some masters in the field cannot do, even though they are "trained." One does not necessarily need to know about tax calculation and payroll because there are always people one can hire or instruct, but it is better that one does, especially when the company is just starting out, and the capital base is rather thin. Not to forget, the computer with the appropriate programs also can be of great benefit. In theory, you do not have to get involved with mathematics, which means a few headaches less.

Some individuals have relationship problems. This means the same: intention and counter intention. You have the idea of how it should work, and your partner has another. Result: problem! You got involved with a person. Ask yourself, did you get involved with a person or with an idea? Perhaps the person cannot think of other ideas and may not agree with yours. If so, then find someone who can think of other ideas and who can agree with the ideas that you are thinking, or just turn the tables. Are you able to think of other ideas?

Usually, it may be easier to change your own ideas before trying to change someone else's because one can make up a bunch of nonsense and pretend that it is important. Therefore, one should evaluate one's ideas in terms of reason, logic and the eight dynamics. It is an important matter when both partners do not evaluate each other's ideas on a common basis because togetherness can never be achieved without this. This inability has led to many relationships falling apart! Of course, you also can be free from it and defend your freedom in terms of a partnership by not having a partnership in the first place, which should not mean that if you have a relationship you do not have to forego personal freedom there. Just as the relationship may be important, the person himself, within the relationship, is also important, which means that the relationship, like the individual himself, has its rights and duties.

But in regard to the human, what is really going on? All too often he is fixated on one thing. He is unable to let go of this one thing and has to have it, which can be observed especially in interpersonal relationships. There, this one person is of importance. Thus, the person himself has a problem, a problem with letting go of a thought and a problem with thinking and allowing another thought. Feeling? Well, this feeling arises from a thought. A feeling is an energy impulse that can be measured. By creating the same feeling in your mind, it dissolves. What I mean by this is that it is the case often enough that the human allows himself to be made a fool because of a feeling. What for? Be the cause about it and turn it off!

Then there are some who have problems with their figure. Well, the person is not in agreement regarding what he or she currently looks like - either too fat or too thin, too little bosom or too much belly. It is likely that the person has too few problems to worry about. When someone has too few problems, he or she chooses something to worry about. A remedy to a problem of course would be to create a problem of the same magnitude, such as imagining that you have no bosom at all, or that your belly would be much bigger. This is how to get the person to be satisfied with what he or she is now, thereby eliminating the problem.

But apart from that, there is actually an idea behind the shape of a body. They are not the genes; these are almost the same from cell to cell. They are like the building blocks of a house, and it is the idea of how the house is supposed to look. However, the normal *homo sapiens** has no direct access to the ideas that determine the shape of the body; therefore, one has to run mental processes. It has already been observed that some can eat like a barn thresher* and not gain a gram of weight, while others just think about food and get fat. In any case, it has been proven that, according to mental processes, the body weight as well as the structure of the body even out. Too thin increases, too fat decreases, and the proportions shift to where they belong.

Problems? Well, they are the things that one causes oneself.

Stress

Some of our fellow human beings already have "stress" when they have to get up at 7:00 A.M. to talk to their employment agent at the employment office. The word stress is used in our society for any situation or activity. Everything is stress!

There is significant difference between the traditional occurrences in everyday life and events that deserve the name stress. So, what is stress? According to the origin of the word, *stress* = deforming force. Stress is a force that acts on something for so long until it breaks.

Life consists of eight dynamics. Every dynamic requires a certain amount of time and money. Time and money are limited resources, and, all too often, we are required to complete tasks that demand more time, money and performance than is available – here one has actual stress!

Stress means that one has lost control. One no longer controls his surroundings. Rather, the surroundings determine what the person should or should not do. The person has to do it because he **cannot** escape from any obligation. The person is under stress (a) when she has to do something against her will, or (b) something happens that she cannot defend herself against.

By mentally finding oneself in a hopeless situation or by actually failing to meet one's obligations, one is under pressure. The pressure is mental pressure. One worries about how the matter will continue. Specifically, two acquaintances come to mind: The owner of a handicraft firm was heavily in debt and had a heart attack. Both day spas of an owner had been failing for some time; this resulted in high debt that eventually led to the owner having a massive stroke.

There seems to be a mechanism that ensures that the stressed person removes himself from circulation. If there is there too much pressure, the person caves in – he gets sick.

It should not matter from what kind of stress one suffers. Stress has a suppressor, something or someone that is stronger than the person, even if it is only imagined! One does not have any stress by having one's surroundings under control or by just having the idea of being in control of one's surroundings. However, the slightest creeping up of a dark idea that things could get out of hand can result in stress. That is why the human has a strong desire for security, be it from a material thing or from his fellow human beings on whom he can rely.

Stress begins with "having" – remember: You have a body. As soon as one has something, one has to take care of it by expending time, money and activity. Ultimately, there is only one form of stress: the will of the person.

The person has stress when:
- He wants to have something and cannot get it.
- He has something, and there is danger that it will be taken away from him.
  He has something and can no longer get rid of it, *also*
- He desperately wants to do something and is prevented from doing it.
- He does something, and there is a danger that it is bad.
- He has done something bad, and he can no longer undo it.

Remedy: Only accept or agree to as much as can be achieved based on one's time, money, qualification and performance, or through the procurement of more money, more time, a higher level of performance and appropriate qualifications alone or with the help of others.

Some people have "stress" because they do not do all of the things that should be done or do not completely finish what they start. Things that are not completed are constantly circling in one's head. At some point, there are so many that one thinks he will lose control. No matter where one looks, no matter what topic is currently being discussed, a thought constantly comes from the back of the head reminding one of what still needs to be done. And this is all because the things were not completed systematically (one after the other).

How can you concentrate on something new when the old stuff continuously keeps going through your head? So, make a "To-Do List." Write everything down and then work through your list systematically according to its importance! You will have less stress!

If you feel like you have a lot of stress, consider the following:
- Converse with others to possibly find a better solution or to gain a different point of view regarding the matter, or
- Take some "Time-Out" in the form of physical activity or other kind of dis-

traction so that you can take some distance from the bustle of thoughts to be able to tackle the matter again later with new vigor.

Stress is a purely mental matter. Stress is when one has lost control over his life! When the person changes his intentions about things, he will no longer have any stress. And yes, the stupid and idle* person will end up having the most stress! I wonder why? Therefore, create an environment that will bring you solutions, not problems!

Acute stress: Serious sudden changes for which a person is not prepared can trigger acute stress. The person can go into a state of shock and temporarily lose his sanity. When someone is under shock, he will no longer react appropriately to his surroundings.

One could say that there is positive or negative stress. Examples of positive stress are winning the lotto or inheriting one million dollars from an unknown uncle in the United States of America. Examples of negative stress are a car accident or the sudden loss of something or someone dear. Nevertheless, stress is stress and can result in a state of shock whether the person sinks into apathy or completely flips out! To overcome shock, the person has to get used to the new reality. Depending on the degree of the shock, this can take some time; however, it can be so severe that the person concerned will suffer from it for the rest of his life.

The psychologist has no appropriate means to handle shock. It is a mental matter that involves the mind, and one will not be able to do anything about it if he does not know about the mind.

In treating shock, the first step is to provide medical attention to the person, if necessary. After that, he should be allowed to rest and remain in an orderly environment away from the accident scenario. Next, the person should re-orient himself in his environment so that he can find reality again. Here, a long walk would be very helpful; however, the person should not ruminate* during the walk. Instead, he should focus his attention on the surroundings and really perceive them (a tree, the edge of the street, yellow flowers, and so forth). It should be a leisurely stroll and not a forced march! If the person is lying in bed, he would alternately focus his attention on the various objects in the room until he feels a bit better.

Mental processes like regression[4] or the running of creative processes, whereby the person repeatedly recalls what has happened in detail when instructed, will dissolve the trauma of the shock. This reduces the mental scarcity and allows the person to let go of what happened. Please keep in mind that creative processes are professional work and require a progressive approach, as well as sensitivity on the part of the practitioner.

War!!!

Are we not living in a beautiful world? You have a place that you think you belong. Everything is beautifully and colorfully painted, and the advertising posters are smiling down on you. You are shown that this world is a beautiful one!

But is it really like that? Well, if you have no money, you will not be able to buy the product that is kindly offered by the poster. And when you finally have the money and have purchased the product, and the product does not perform as promised, you either want your money back or a decent product!

I witnessed how two of my closest friends got into each other's hair when it came to the decision to fill another job in the same company with one of them that included a salary increase. The friendship broke apart! Friendships also fail because, suddenly, the opposite sex played a major role. Or observe the family that breaks apart when it comes to inheritance. Prior to that, it was still one unit that went through thick and thin together!

Every day, people around you greet and smile at you, but what do you think of all that is being whispered behind your back? Generally, the individual is too cowardly to really tell you to your face what he thinks. At my grandmother's golden wedding anniversary, I asked her what it was like to be married for 50 years. She replied, "Yes, 50 years of war!" From my observation, I can only say, "Even in marriage, one has to fight for one's interests, and, by not doing so, one "loses one's life."

When going to court with your lawyer because you believe that you have been wronged, you will likely leave the courtroom astonished, disbelieving what had gone on in there. The opposing party's attorney invented a fairy tale about what action you could have taken to avoid the harm done and, only for one reason, because you were there! In the end, the court offers you a settlement*, and you are made to pay for some of the damage yourself.

It is all the harder in the business world. Larger companies run their own law firm with a bevy* of lawyers to defend themselves or to implement strategies to appease or incapacitate the "competitors in the market." Ultimately, the millions that flow into the quarrels are capital wisely invested. Witness the two small plastering companies that are based in the same town, where the bosses are often at odds. The company worker there can never do a work-related personal favor for any villager because this would be considered illicit* work, and, once the boss found out, he would go on the warpath if his jobs were taken away, no matter how small!

Actually, you are all alone in the world. You always will have to represent your views in front of your fellow human beings, work colleagues, friends and life partner, and you seldom find someone who sees things exactly as you see them. The feeling of personal strength and the feeling of having value in this world arises from your ability to do things right, which means that you are in the right. By constantly making mistakes and constantly being told how very wrong you are, your confidence will dry up*, leaving you to think that you no longer have value.

You will stop thinking for yourself, and you will stop taking responsibility for yourself and for your world. You will stop living your life because you stopped attempting to try to be in the right because you did not defend your right and allowed it to be taken from you. You have become a puppet!

So be capable and be happy! To be happy in this world means to make no or only minor mistakes. Do not go completely on the defensive* when you have made a blunder*. After all, you were the one who did anything at all, and only the one who does not do anything cannot do anything wrong. This is the biggest mistake. Remember: By not doing anything, you will get nowhere! Mistakes can be stamped out*, and things can be repaired. Recognizing a mistake means that it will be better the next time around.

No one will be able to do everything correctly, because there are also such things as inclinations and taste. What is good for one does not necessarily have to be good for the other. But you will find out one thing, the more capable you are, the happier you will be!

Like my mentor writes at the beginning of the advanced lectures, "When Mrs. Cuddle Cakes comes to us to be trained, transform any wandering doubt in her eyes into a firm determined shine, and she will win, and all of us will win. Adapt to her, and we will all die a little." The right training attitude is "Now we are going to make you a capable person, no matter what happens. We would rather have you dead than incapable." It is a tough universe. The social coating makes it appear mild. But only the tigers survive, and even they have a hard time."

Well then, keep your mind awake and sharpen your knives, and do not think that everything will work without any quarrels in this world. It is war, even if only subliminally. War? Too often the human being demonstrates his inability to recognize right and wrong and is unable to come to an amicable* agreement. For this reason, laws have to be devised to patronize the other, and weapons are used to kill the other because no one is able to rethink their own thoughts anew!

Privacy

From where does one get good thought impulses, and what does one do with them? Well, thoughts, among other things, serve to help one understand oneself, one's fellow human being and life. They allow individuals to get by in life without starting a war with another. One is confronted with war all the time, sometimes with and sometimes without weapons and sometimes more or less violently. One only has peace at the cemetery. As Plato* proclaimed, **"Only the dead have seen the end of war!"**

Thought impulses. How often does one have to move back and forth in one's spiritual world until one becomes flexible, loses one's mental barriers, and the meaning of words is no longer crushing? Well, I am happy about everyone who stands up to me and demonstrates that there is also another point of view on a matter. Ultimately, the question then arises, "What is best to use, which piece of knowledge is valid, and are we already back to right and wrong again?" Oh well, it is just the illness of the human being! How about being free or captive? Where and when is the human really free? What about privacy?

Here is the original meaning: From Latin, *privatus* – personal, for itself, freed (from public duties, responsibility, and so on), not princely, imperial or state, to *privus* – existing for itself, individually, free from.

Private. Some do not seem to fully understand the meaning of it. It means that one is free from something and that one has the right to have or not to have something. However, this is not the case in professional life or as a holder of public office, where one often has to submit to survive.

It is important to have in the back of one's mind the concept that professional life is professional life and that the whole private sphere begins at 8:00 P.M. and, as far as I am concerned, ends at 9:00 A.M. During this time, someone else's business or other concerns no longer belong, unless it has been agreed to beforehand! Hence, the front door seems to be the last bastion* of personal freedom to a place where one can decide to relax or to develop personally, keeping the customs and traditions in the corner of one's eye. It is difficult to turn down a surprise visit without upsetting the other a little.

But what does it look like behind the front door? Again, no freedom! There is a system of order and cleanliness to a greater or lesser extent. Even in private, one is absorbed in the rules of society or submits to a system of one's own order. This is inevitable because, otherwise, you would never find anything and would always be searching. Over time, enough things have been accumulated that are in need of organization.

If you neglect your children, they are taken from you. If you are not kind to your wife, you will soon find that she has left you. As you can see, even the private sector is regulated. Violating these rules will result in yellow or red cards or time penalties. If you have collected enough cards, you are excluded from the game because, eventually, there are no more players with whom to play!

Rules and predictability also have some benefit. You do not like it when you do not know what is going on and on what you can orient yourself. Not having this information makes one insecure and unstable and results in confusing states that stand in the way of a happy and content existence. There seem to be a few laws that make the human tick: order and aesthetics*! When things do not correspond to these, he does not seem to like them because, generally, the human likes things when there is something that he can admire about them. Look around yourself in your world, and you will find that there is at least something about your things that pleases you.

So, if you cannot be free, make it a game and see that you have fun with it. Why else should you have lived?

P.S. As long as you are in this universe, you will never really be private!

Getting Something Done! – The Power of the Second Person –

I remember a construction site that I was still working on in the evening. It was around 10:30 P.M., and I was dog tired; I had no more energy and was about to drop everything. Actually, there was not much left to do, maybe another thirty minutes, but I just could not finish the job, and my morale was at rock bottom.

Then I remembered a foundation of my studies in which I learned that the practitioner and the treated are stronger than the mind (idea) of the treated. This is also the reason, among other things, why two people should be present to run mental processes with one person in command who leads and ensures that the other person does not give up or go astray. Using the vernacular*, one would say, "Vanquish the inner temptation." So, I called Stefan, my boss and friend at the time, and asked him if he could come by to help me boost my morale. He actually came late that evening, and his presence provided enough drive for me to finish the work. ☺

Indeed, it seems that the person is usually subject to the weaker self; the idea from the mind is stronger than the person's will. I once heard someone say that it is not the lack of orders that is the downfall of sole proprietorships, but the inability to pull oneself together to maintain self-discipline. It seems that someone has to be present to whom one seems to owe something, best of all someone who stands above one in the form of a foreman or a boss. This idea of obligation to one's superior is indeed what drives the individual to demonstrate virtues that enable one to make and to fulfill obligations.

This is the reason why some people only manage to exercise by joining a community or going to a gym. Of course, the matter will turn into a disaster when all are of the opinion that nothing will get done today. Therefore, a superordinate person is needed who maintains an idea and enforces it. Should he fail to implement the idea, all will fail. A real boss is the only guarantee that things will work, because if he does not succeed, the company will perish.

This reminds of the daughter of my former schoolmate Jörg. She constantly kept bringing home bad grades. Jörg took the time and practiced with his daughter. Lo and behold, after some time, she only received A's and B's. Being good at something is seldom a lack of ability; it requires someone who leads and who demonstrates little indulgence in leading. When one begins to agree with the other's whining, both lose, but a good coach knows what works and what does not. And since one cannot kick oneself in the behind, someone has to be there to do it!

Why cannot the person just get the stuff done? Here the question would be, "What is he not confronting? By starting to point out the matter which is to be done, the person concerned begins to justify his actions to himself by saying such things as: "I have no time; it's too difficult; I have other things to do; I want to have my free time; I do not understand it; I cannot do it; it's too much, and so on. Or he attacks you directly, "First sweep in front of your own door; your so and so are not that much better; what actually became of so and so, and the like."

All too often it gets personal, "You are too stupid for ... ." Objectivity is lost, and one no longer refers to one matter exactly. One indulges in generalizations, and if one asks, "Who exactly said that?" or "What exactly was said?" too often the other person owes an answer. Generalizations are now the final act against defeat when trying to fight the other.

Well, all of this talk is preventing things getting done! How much easier it would be to sit down and think about whether the matter is important and if it should be done in a timely manner. The person concerned should think in terms of solutions, instead of justifying or even attacking.

It is complete disaster for a weak person when he gets involved with a weaker one. The weaker derives his energy from the stronger, and the stronger has to muster energy to get the weaker to do something. If the stronger one stops putting energy into it in the form of, "Now do it!", or "That is still not done!", things will not get done. The weaker one should pull himself together and stop turning against the other. He should recognize himself and be happy that the other is taking care of him! If he does not, then both of them will lose because the mess around them will get bigger.

And yes, not getting something done, is just the thought that keeps the person from doing it!

Getting One's Own Stuff Done
Yes, indeed: **When wanting things to get done, one has to take care of them oneself, so that they get done!**

As a rule, pending tasks should be completed in a very specific way. The letter should be written in a certain way and be sent to arrive before the deadline. But what does the husband do? "Woman, could you also mail this letter for me?" Well, she takes it along, puts it into her car and drives it around for three days. Result: A missed deadline and preprogrammed problems and anger.

Or: "Could you just ..." This is how one brings the instructed person out of his rhythm and out of his plan. Authorities are now trying to achieve a well-functioning procedure by defining areas of jurisdiction, whereby everyone has an area that he must regulate. Well, why not also do this in the private sector? People take care of their own stuff that way. This way one cannot blame the other for making a mistake.

Or: "Honey, would you get me a beer?" This question alone pressures one to act, because the one being asked may want the other to do a favor for her in the future. It is better to operate on one level where one takes care of the things that concern oneself. Of course, in a household, one holds things in common, like laundry or other house and gardening work, but even this can be settled fairly by at least talking about it.

What about doing something for someone else or giving a recommendation? One thing is certain, when things go wrong, you are the culprit! Of course, one can give one tip or another, but in the same breath one should point out that, while it worked well for oneself, it cannot be assured that it will work for the other. Everyone should take care of his own affairs, read the documents themselves and deal with things themselves. I mean, one should know about one's own things! What will happen when the other person, who took care of matters, is no longer there? Everyone should be able to manage one's own life.

Getting one's own things done? Do not borrow any tools or other equipment from your acquaintances! Get your own things. How quickly does something break, get damaged, or is not clean when it is returned! You also never know in what condition the equipment was borrowed. If these items already had outlived their usefulness, they can quickly break. So you pay twice, once for the old tool that broke and for a new one because the work has not yet been completed.

To borrow something means to owe someone something. In short, with the use of other people's goods, the relationship with them is also at stake!

And yes: **Ingratitude is the salary of the world!**

Communication – The Key to the World

As previously mentioned, your world consists of the eight dynamics, and existence always has something to do with communication. For example, if you want something from Peter, you will want to talk to him, unless you are a thief and steal it.

When someone caused an automobile accident on the road, it could be said that he had insufficient communication* with the road. He did not understand something, and, thereupon, acted wrongly, and it happened.

Communication is not only about talking but, above all, about listening and **understanding**. The components of communication are affinity*, reality and, of course, language – even the deaf and mute have a language! Communication usually works like this: The communicator perceives, understands and acts. Then the person opposite perceives, understands and acts. If there is no action or answer in this cycle, the communicator will get an "answer hunger," because he is not satisfied and, after a while, will be disgruntled*. An example of proper communication: Mother, "Do you want milk?" Child, "Yes." Mother, "Very well."

Likewise, in baseball: The pitcher throws the ball to the batter, who tries to hit the ball with his bat. Thus, we have intention and attention – cause, distance and effect. One can have a game by being in communication.

If you do not like someone, you do not want to talk to him either. When taking a closer look, you will find that if you like someone you have things in common, a common reality that is talked about. The more common reality, the more communication, the more affinity – one leans towards the other. You have someone with whom you get along! But beware! To agree with everything and to do what others do, does not seem authentic*, making you a follower, a marionette*!

An example from an Opel Manta meeting in Germany: George walks through the rows of highly polished and "souped-up" cars, when he sees a car standing there that looks almost like his. It even has the same rims and, "Oh no!", the same exhaust system. George talks to the guy who is standing there. His name is Frank, and he is the owner of the car. "Hey, what did you pay for the exhaust system?" Hence, a conversation develops, and George finds out that, like himself, Frank is a New York Yankees fan and goes fishing when he wants to be left in peace. Result: friends for life.

Later on, when Frank gets married, stops fishing, sells his Manta and takes weekend excursions with his family, instead of going to ballgames, the friendship suffers greatly. Now one probably does not understand the other anymore because previously everything was different.

As you can see, you can make an effort to communicate; you just have to speak to someone. In other words, initiate the conversation. Find something about the person and talk to him about it, such as, "Nice shoes. I want to gift something like this to my sister, but I have no idea where to buy them."

When someone acts stupidly when being spoken to, the person simply shows what he or she is! Very good, you now know how he or she is and can rest assured that this is nothing you need to have!!! Incidentally, it is an extremely bad state of affairs when one is fixated on having something. It is always the personal mishmash* that prevents the human being from being "free."

Having a Conversation

Unfortunately, I am not very well read when it comes to communication. I mean, there are many different forms that have been worked out scientifically, but the "boys" turn a fly into an elephant. Why should I contribute to the tons of material on a topic when there is not much to say about it, except for a few basics that are usually not conclusively worked out!

Although I may not consider myself being well-read, I may have read a little more than Victoria Beckham*. As I recently saw on the Internet, she has not read a single book, causing some to question her intellect. However, I think that books read are not an indicator of high intellect. When I look at an acquaintance of mine, I hardly believe that he has the time to read books. A talented craftsman with a family, he successfully runs a company, doing so without any training. On the other hand, there are scholars who cannot drive a nail into the wall and who also demonstrate extreme difficulties with regard to living in society. Why is this so? Ultimately, it is all about how one finds one's way through life.

Nowadays, the mind gets more corrupt through reading than educated, as words are usually never looked up, and the quality of the reading material leaves a lot to be desired. However, here I must say that without reading, I never would have gotten to where I am now; it just depends on what one reads.

The human often speaks of "a common sense," except that he does not possess it. It would be better if he had no mind at all and would only use his eyes to see instead of thinking what the world is about. I mean, he can easily be talked into or made to believe of all sorts of things. For example, it is said that someone demonstrates an unwillingness to communicate by crossing his arms or legs. Of course, no one would even consider that this contributes to a more comfortable sitting position or that the woman simply feels more elegant by doing this. This on the subject of "common sense!"

Actually, I wanted to use the title called "communication," but I already have it; therefore, this article simply serves as an extension of "communication" and "language." So, what actually is the basic foundation of communication? Some believe that it is the word or the language because communication usually is associated with talking. Well, there are people who do not speak a word and get along very well!

Communication comes from Latin *communis* = common; this is the basic foundation: to have something in common. For example, when someone speaks Chinese to you, you do not understand one word, hence no communication and nothing in common, unless you are Chinese yourself or know the language.

The modern world speaks of rhetoric*, dialectic*, eloquence* and transforms this simple matter of communication into a very difficult scientific one. This most important basis of communication should now be followed if one wants to have successful conversations. Before one word has even been spoken, all negotiations may have failed already if one does not know and does not heed the customs and traditions of the other person.

Here, in the Western world, one dresses appropriately for the occasion and greets one another with a handshake. This is customary for men in Germany. In Italy or in Russia, one hugs one another and gives the other a faint kiss on the cheek, even among men. One demonstrates respect one shows manners* and respects customs and traditions. Failure to do so can create the appearance of arrogance and as is known from the *Bible*: Arrogance comes before the fall! If one does not know the customs and traditions, one should at least be polite and reserved and behave like the others, unless one is prompted to do something specific.

The next important point is attention. One should not be distracted and should listen to what the other has to say. When he has finished with his statement, he should confirm that with an "ok," or turn to the topic. Not paying attention to the other person or showing him that the communication sent has arrived, is very impolite and may influence the further course of the conversation.

Here, I would like to mention that it is important to greet one's neighbors and fellow human beings, as well as to be friendly and, in the best case, to offer a little time. By greeting, one shows that one notices the other person and is not arrogant, which the other person is likely to think immediately when one does not offer a greeting.

Furthermore, one should adapt to the diction of the other. Diction means something like choice of words, which is another point that one can have in common. This carries a lot of weight in building sympathy, enabling one to be understood.

A very human indication during the course of conversation is the facial expression, meaning what can be seen on the face of the other person. I mean, you can see very clearly if someone is cheerful or annoyed, so realize this and act accordingly. One could ask, for example, what is wrong, not suitable, or disturbing to the others? One should change the subject when noticing that the other has nothing to say. Communication control is done with questions. The more information one has about the other, the more targeted communication can be established. Keep in mind that it is everyone's decision whether or not to have communication. If someone does not want to talk to you, accept that. Likewise, you have to recognize the point of being intrusive*, so try to avoid it. If you have a pleasant conversation with the person opposite, he will talk to you again.

A person feels understood when you take the idea that he conveys to you through his words. One does not have to broaden one's opinion directly, just question what exactly he means by the expressed idea and how he relates to it. One can incorporate the other's idea into the answer.

For example, if the person opposite tells you that he bumped his knee, do not tell him in the same breath that the same thing happened to you three days ago. Instead, ask him how it happened and let him tell you about it. It is often the case that the other person "opens a barrel" with his first words, only with the difference that the content oozes out. By stopping the whole matter with an inappropriate comment or personal experience, you will not have any successful communication. Therefore, "let the barrel run empty." True listening is perhaps an art, and it is remarkable to note that one can hardly find anyone who really listens.

Emotions can be reduced to some extent by having someone who simply listens to what one closely sees in one's mind. By looking at it and communicating, one releases oneself from a fixed mindset and can again breathe freely, allowing the person to direct his attention freely afterwards. This from my time as a practitioner, "The way out is the way through!" It also should be mentioned here that it is definitely worth taking a sensible communication course that teaches one of how to keep one's own "mishmash" under control while communicating and how to encourage the person opposite to continue talking, unless it is necessary to stop him if he just babbles without meaning. Communication also means to get one's own questions answered and not to deviate.

Success in life has a lot to do with communication because the togetherness always is a kind of partnership, be it as a life companion, a boss or a subordinate. Communication is the bond of this partnership. Thus, if communication is broken, the partnership will also break. Just consider a divorce, which can be your ruin, costing tens of thousands of dollars. The same applies for maintaining and keeping a place of employment. How to approach the matter is always related to the form of communication. Do not shy away from investing in yourself.

Prior to starting a conversation, one should have a concept of how to proceed and what goal one wants to achieve. In the case of particularly important discussions, one should have practiced beforehand in a role-play in which the trainer tries to depict the actual situation.

Let us say that you are on a train trip. Opposite from you, there is a young lady whom you would like to get to know – this text is not intended to be a comprehensive guide. As a rule, people identify very strongly with what they wear in the sense that it should be presentable. Shoes, brand-name clothing or jewelry can represent something special for the person wearing them. In this way, one can start a conversation by noticing what is special about the person. For example, "Those are nice shoes. I once saw a similar style in Italy. Have you been there before?" It remains to be seen whether the lady will respond to the communication.

With this in mind, one should be skilled enough to ask general questions without coming straight to the point. Perhaps one could tell a funny story about what one has already experienced to break the ice and brighten up the atmosphere. With knowledge about the professional activity, favorite books and hobbies of the person opposite, one will quickly have an insight into the spiritual horizon of the other and maybe find something that one has in common or can have in common. Maybe the other is engaged in something that one always wanted to know more about.

By the way, one more small matter. There is a very human attribute that will open doors that even the highest IQ cannot open: charm. Charm means something like grace, sweetness or loveliness. The human being will never bother to accumulate things around himself that he does not like. Therefore, this is the reverse conclusion. Constant smiling is inappropriate; however, showing an accommodating smile at the right moment is indeed the key to the door!

Remember, the outer appearance is an important factor. Your face will likely transform into a grimace* when a big fat hag* gives you an inviting wink of the eye. Be smart!

P.S. In conclusion, I would like to say that it is rare to have an interesting conversation because it is up to each individual whether it will continue to be so.

The Date

Now it counts. The first moment is often decisive. Your outer appearance has to be right. Shaved, hair styled or cut, clean clothing – you of course as well. Should you use a deodorant or perfume, make sure that it does not seem obtrusive. Keep in mind that if her ex used the same perfume, then you are likely to bring back bad memories. Be on time because it is a sign that the date is important to you. If you cannot come in your car, tell her that and the reason why. Be truthful and responsible. Show that you can be polite and wear your Sunday smile ☺.

If you find the first impression went really well, use a little gimmick* – something special. For example, offer a small piece of wrapped chocolate with a lovely note that says, "A sweet for the sweet." This gesture makes an impression and shows your commitment. If you meet at a coffee shop, you are not required to pay the bill.

Incidentally, I often appeared so trustworthy on the phone that the first date took place at the lady's home. I also managed to invite myself to dinner at the lady's home on my first date. I just suggested that we cook something together. I brought the ingredients, she cooked, and I assisted as best I could. It was fun. This, by the way, is better than sitting across from one another in a café. Of course, meeting for a walk or going window shopping is also possible. Be somewhat inventive in this because it makes for a relaxed atmosphere.

Should you have the idea that it possibly will not work out with the lady because you do not like her, and so forth, tell her that. If it is the other way around, pull yourself together and leave her alone.

Remember, there are many fish in the ocean.

When you are finally full of euphoria* because you found someone with whom it could work out, hold back somewhat with your phone calls and visits. Try to turn the whole thing around, so that she can take care of you as well. Try not to push because pressure results in counter pressure. Your tactic should be reaching out and pulling back. Remember:

- **Try not to do something to others that you do not want to experience yourself** (LRH).
- **Try to treat others as you would like them to treat you** (LRH).

The Right One

"True Love!" How fortunate! One has butterflies in one's stomach, the world appears friendlier with its colors, and the sun shines in new splendor. One gets up in good spirits in the morning and faces the day with great motivation. No job seems too difficult and no problem too big. The future is full of hope! There is only one thing that inspires the human that much: love!

On the other hand, there is a crash landing when one loses a loved one. Existence sinks into a melancholy* gray, all hope is lost, and life no longer has any meaning.

So, what exactly happens to the human being? From what deep morass* is the human pulled out by the feeling of love? How deep has the human sunk spiritually that there is a feeling that makes him blossom so? The human is overwhelmed by his past. He is degraded to a spectator and often just an incompetent actor. Some even are willing to take their own lives for love. What nonsense. At most, one can deprive oneself of one's body but to take a life is impossible. Life is you, yourself and not the body. At most, you can give "life" to the body because you are the one who experiences existence. You feel the sun's rays on your skin, the pain when the little toe hits the table leg and the feeling of love, which originates from somewhere. To perceive means to receive the impulses of the environment.

This is probably a tooth that has to be extracted from some. "True love" means to be overwhelmed by a feeling, a feeling that is so strong that one loses his senses but only because one has long lost one's real strength. "True love" means chasing after one's own imagination. Before one begins a relationship, one has a dream: an idea of what the relationship should be like. When love for a person ignites, one reflects upon one's dream. One probably no longer notices the person opposite with his or her mistakes, characteristics and idiosyncrasies because one only has this feeling and one's dream! Hence the saying: **Love is blind!**

Have you ever seen a puppy when his owners come home? The dog can be so exuberant* in his joy that he lets go of everything and sometimes even urinating on the floor.

To love means to feel a feeling. This feeling is sent from the "soul." The soul is an entity. It is the mind of cows, dogs, cats ... of animals. More precisely, the soul is the ruler of the organism. The soul gives the organism the impulse to survive for the intake of food and reproduction. From a truly technical point of view, it operates on a coarser level than you (spirit). Since you are in a body, you can feel the soul's impulses. You are in the head, and the soul is in the stomach. This is why one has a tingling sensation when one is in love. Technically, the feeling of love is a flow of energy on a certain wavelength, a weak electric current. There are mental processes related to this energy phenomenon. After all, you are a spiritual being that thinks in images of weak electrical energy, and thus you can encounter any kind of energy impulse in a certain way.

Feeling "love" is a beautiful thing; there is nothing wrong with it. However, a lot is wrong with it when one perishes from this energy impulse! Thus, men look after women and women after men. If this were not the case, the days of the human race would long be numbered. In the animal kingdom, there is not much fuss about the matter of procreation*. Only the human turns it into a huge farce* among his own kind and complicates this matter with jealousy and moral values that he himself considers to be good. And even those who preach about it do not adhere to it!

One is dealing with subtle* thinking and sensitive beings, and, in that sense, one should be careful. The intended moral rules actually aid in self-protection.

Thus, one could say that love is a purely psychological matter. Observe for yourself: "Love at first sight." You see the other for the first time and already have this sensation. You have fallen "in love" with the body of the other person, the person himself, but you do not even know his essence. "Knowing someone" is a matter in itself.

The human does not know himself! There are situations in which he reacts in a certain way that he is not familiar with at all. Subsequently, he apologizes for his misconduct. The human mind is messed up! "A relationship" does not fail because of love but because of the human's crazy mind and the fact that he does not have a sensible manual on "how to get along" with his contemporaries. Even the old adage asserted by George Bernard Shaw*, "Do not do unto others as you would that they should do unto you" does not work if the person has missed parameters* and misconceptions about right and wrong. No wonder, only a genius will write a brilliant book, and a madman will proclaim only madness, no matter how sophisticated he may be. Just deal with the tax law and you will know what I am talking about. This is likewise true for the healing methods of psychiatry and medicine, as well as for training and the self-consuming democracies of the 21st century.

The Odyssey* in the matter of the human is that unreason does not recognize reason and, consequently, does not acknowledge it. Unreason is unreason, and this is the majority of humanity.

The right one? Well, are you the right one for him? The human is what he is. Is your thought the right one? Are you actually looking at the human in front of you and not at your thoughts?! It is likely the human can never be as complete as his thoughts.

The right one: Where does one find him? You can find him where your thoughts are also circling. The right one is the right one when one has a common approach and cherishes common interests, which does not mean that one cannot find common interests later in the relationship! Just falling in love and having sex is not a problem. As a friend of mine once said, "When love is made of wine, it lasts like wine, only one night." Just like, "love at first sight," which one only loves one another because of love, this kind of love is not a bond for life. Then when you find him, tell him you love him and that every day without him is a lost day. How else will he know how much you care about him if you do not do this?

Love? Is this not just self-interest, personal sensation, or sexual satisfaction? How much space do you give the other? How much are you really there for the other?

Being in love? What is the greater sensation? To be happy that the other is there or the pain of separation, the uncertainty of seeing him again and the worries when he is gone? One could say that by being in love, one is rarely happy. But to feel the happiness and to lay in each other's arms outweighs everything! Yes, that's how it is; the human builds his own prison!

Unhappily in love*? Not wanting to hurt the other? This will not fail to happen! It is probable that nowhere have there been more wounds inflicted than on the battlefield of love. More than in all wars combined, given that everyone has likely suffered losses in love at least once.

Flirting means giving the other a sign that one wants to enter into a love affair with the other. Remember, only do it if you really mean it! And reject it if you do not want it or already have a partner. This way, you can avoid a lot of heartache, unnecessary contacts and calls. Hold back your affection and put it to full use for what you want.

Lovesickness? Yes, there is confusion in human existence! Basically, the human has the natural impulse and also the desire to fall in love because he wants to have this thing called love.

Lovesickness arises from rejected love. One wants to give one's love to the other, but the other rejects it. There may be several reasons for that:

1. One fell in love unhappily, one is not his type, the other is already taken, or
2. The relationship fell apart, and each goes his or her separate ways, even though one still has feelings for the other.

In any case, the problem is: One is stuck in a mess! And this feeling cannot simply be turned off. The fact is that one is stuck in the past with one's thoughts. You first had to get to know the other person before you could develop feelings for him. Then one either made love, and it fell apart, or one would very much love to love the other. This, however, remains denied, from which the grief arises. You catch yourself actually looking at a picture from the past that you would like to have realized in the present.

Although it is easy to dwell in the past, now you must force yourself to bring your thoughts into the present and to align them there with what you can still have. Some talk about distracting oneself. No, it is not a distraction; it is the realigning of your thoughts! However, you can focus your thoughts by concentrating on something, like burying yourself in a professional activity or sports or by participating in a club.

It is even better if you just start searching for a new partner. There are millions looking for a partnership! And do not cry to the new partner about what happened to you because this is poison for a fresh start. After all, how would you feel if you kept hearing from your new partner that he was thinking of someone else?

Focus on the new partner and make an effort to get to know him without comparing him to the old one! Keep in mind, if you do not detach your thoughts from the old and direct them to the new partner, you will suffer setbacks. You have to work on letting go. This means no more calling and no more meeting because it will only make it worse!

"True love" is that what it is: a dream! Maybe you think like me that it should be for eternity when you enter into a relationship with someone, just like the dream you dream. Now who says that dreams cannot be lived? Just maybe at some point it will be time to wake up and dream another dream!

You may be thinking, "Oh, if I just had not read all of this!" Well, things are as there are. It is up to you to understand yourself. When you understand things for yourself, nobody will be able to fool you any longer.

P.S. And in this theater is the human being stuck. He no longer sees the game as a game but turns everything into a deadly serious matter.

Sex

Sexuality in regard to life is as important as eating and drinking because it is the only guarantee for the continued existence of the human race. The human finds that sex has a great effect in the sense that he can be manipulated through sex and that out of this comes the desire to do things that one would not do out of pure mind. This desire for the other can be so strong that dignity, decency, rules and law can lose their validity and no longer be observed. To somehow slow this down, the human makes sex bad. In the case of the Catholic Church, it is even forbidden with the edict of celibacy* although the "Boss" proclaims in his book, "Beget and multiply!"

The politician speaks about moral values: Pornography must be forbidden and the brothels banned from the city, only to find him there later on. He makes sexuality bad, and even the youth must be protected from it. I mean, he did not understand something! If you want to become a politician in this society, you have practically lost if people can accuse you of immoral behavior. "Is he running for the party? He used to be together with Lissy, the local madam*." He is morally not impeccable having had the wrong contact in his youth. Getting rid of an uncomfortable person? Just accuse him or her of having an affair!

Thus, it is hammered into the youth that sex is a bad thing. What is so bad about it? Peter falls in love, enjoys himself with his girlfriend, and she cheats on him with another. The relationship fails. Peter is hurt, and, to make matters worse, he has to argue about a questionable paternity. Yes, this hurt, and there were losses and a lot of trouble. But what does one have to do with the other? Just because a relationship was unhappy, sex does not have to be bad after all. The child from this relationship is delighted to be here and goes its way.

Is it the responsibility that one has towards the child? Perhaps this hits the nail on the head by telling someone to take responsibility when he seeks distance. Hit and run, if you understand.

Thomas is now a father. We exchanged a few words about the matter, and he told me that he also had to hear that sex was a bad thing. He is now 41 and takes care of the baby. "If I had become a father at the age of 20, it would have been so," he said. "Life goes on even under these circumstances, and it has its nice sides!"

My mentor writes in his books that people in the former Roman Empire were employed in their early teens and married at the beginning of sexual maturity, which is the natural development. People today think they know better and violate a natural process, enacting laws and making all kinds of fuss about this matter.

The human being has the impulse to reproduce in a natural way. After all, sexuality is part of the body. For some parents, having the child masturbate seems close to a tragedy. It is bad ... bad ... bad. The child then feels bad about it as well and is ashamed. The result is a sexually repressed adult whose relationship then falls apart when he fails in sexual terms with his partner. He cannot satisfy her.

Satisfaction means to have one's peace. The sexual impulse affects the person, and the person wants to have peace just like when one hungers, thirsts or freezes. During puberty, the human discovers his sexual emotional world and satisfies the impulse that arises there. One develops a desire for the opposite sex and realizes that when one is touched by the other in the sexually-oriented areas, the sensations are much more intense, and the satisfaction is higher. My God. It is just a body, and the body is designed accordingly, basta*! There is no right or wrong; only the human invents a moral for it –messed up mind!

An ex-girlfriend of mine believed, "Whatever is fun, is allowed." Therefore, from a sexual point of view, things are right to do that satisfy the other and enable him to enjoy his lust. So, ask him what he wants and what excites him the most. Nobody likes a boring relationship!

When I asked her how many times she thought about sex, she replied, "Always!" If the sexual desire for the other is asleep, the relationship is at risk. The sexual impulse is still present; it is something that one cannot easily turn off. You stop starving when you have eaten!

Furthermore, sexuality is a part of quality of life. How would you react when all you get in your life is poor quality while knowing that there is something better? Living a beautiful life has something to do with the quality of it, which is good or bad. As a rule, poor quality cannot be kept well.

There is a bit of confusion concerning love and sex. One hears about "making love," that is to have sex. One thing should be clear to everyone: Love arises out of the sexual impulse. Love is the feeling that one carries in oneself, which leads to sexuality, an established mechanism in the human being. Some people fall in love at first sight, while others develop this feeling over time, and some only realize the love for the other when he is no longer there.

There are a couple of key points to turning on this mechanism. This is the reason why woman behave towards men as they do and dress as they dress. It boils down to sexuality, to have an effect on the other, to please or even to be loved. It is also sufficient to turn the other on with words because words also activate this impulse. It is the thoughts that go through one's head. Thus, men look at women and women look at men. The impulse to sexuality is almost omnipresent*. In any case, in this society with its moral rules, one can save oneself a lot of trouble by being monogamous*.

Being jealous and almost freaking out when your partner looks at another is inappropriate. This was only due to an impulse, and it may include a thought or two. However, one decides to do it or not to do it, but if one is in a bad relationship, one seriously has to consider whether the partner is actually flirting with someone else. Or is it the wrong partner after all? However, staring at the other is a bit tactless. Being looked at may be flattering, but God forbid one's own partner looks at another. Then the tolerance limit is often reached quickly.

He has only one thing in mind ... of course it is going in that direction, and it is not bad! Or why do you maintain sexual relations with the opposite sex? Imagine if your partner had no sex organs and would not like physical contact, not even cuddling or hugging!

Indeed, what is fulfilling is having sex with a human being whom one loves. Mere sex is not a real bond, which is so important for a future family. True love is a strong bond; however, it may be very fickle* when one breaks its rules!

Sex is a peculiar matter to the human being, and he should be free in that regard. It is better for the bachelor to amuse himself in the brothel or to educate himself with pornography, rather than to rape a woman. So, in my opinion, the sexually uptight husband who cheats on his wife ultimately became a victim of those in this society who made sex bad. And indeed, it is so that society makes itself a victim, complicating its own existence by banishing a natural matter with naturalness!

Being ashamed to face the other naked? Well, nobody is perfect! And you really do not have to be ashamed of yourself! Teenagers are reading Bravo* and everyone has probably seen pornos*! One knows how the other looks naked.

Awesome sex? It is not intercourse per se. One has awesome sex when one really turns the other on, and he can barely wait to be touched. In fact, it is the foreplay that makes the whole thing worthwhile. After all, the word excite does not exist for nothing. This means, among other things, that one challenges something and that the other prepares for it. One does not excite the other simply by grasping him directly between his legs or by fumbling awkwardly under the sweater. One approaches the whole thing and then withdraws again.

The Desire to Be the Effect

Well, to experience something in life means to be an effect. One is the effect of something by experiencing things with one's senses because it is the perception that affects one.

Let us take sex for example. To have sex is to want the pleasant sensations that one receives. However, an action must take place to feel the feeling, so there has to be a cause. It is like that in the partnership in which one wishes to be the effect of one's partner. However, some seem to forget that one also can be a cause, whereby a healthy and functioning relationship consists of equal parts of effect and cause. Some are only an effect in the partnership and let things happen without taking responsibility themselves because responsibility has something to do with causation, that is to be responsible for the consequences.

Then there is the irrational attitude, which implies that if one wants to be effective during sex, one should also keep still in everyday situations. Perhaps the looming loss also resonates that if one rebelled and tried to assert one's opinion and will that one would lose love. How deep has one sunk? Has one become a slave to an effect? This is one of the reasons why sex is bad. The invitation to sensation also has negative side effects such as venereal diseases or an unwanted child. These are the things that one does not want to have as a result of sex, whereby the positive and negative phenomena are being lumped together and the whole topic made bad. Then there are also the envious, those who begrudge one the things one has. Often nothing good comes out of their mouth.

Interest in something means the desire to be an effect. One will only experience a fulfilling and happy existence by being a cause and allowing an effect. For example, you want to ride a motorcycle. You are in the cause position in your decision to buy the motorcycle. You come into an effect position when it comes to maintaining the motorbike, even when it comes to the joyful part of riding the motorbike. You decide to accelerate and lean into the curve, but, at the same time, you experience the effect of the occurring forces and the limits of physics. And it is precisely this relationship between cause and effect that gives you pleasure because you see that you are in control of the motorcycle. However, the loss of control is pain, the opposite of joy, and this is the effect that you do not want to experience while riding a motorcycle!

Education and upbringing have a lot to do with effect in this culture. Sitting in the classroom or listening to the rebuke* of the elderly put you in an effect position. Of course, one first has to be an effect in the learning process to absorb the data. However, too often the flow in the other direction is lacking, and this is the establishment of a cause. One will only then master the events of life when one has learned to deal with ideas. Every situation has its own characteristics, and one has to adapt one's own ideas to it, and, to get the best out of it, this requires independent thinking. Thus, successful training would enable the student to be a creative thinker. Making the learner fully effective by only being allowed to do exactly what he is told is the gateway to crime. It does not imply any responsibility, independent thinking or doing, which opens the door to complete incapacity.

Matter is the effect of the mind. The mind has the ability to think creatively. The carpenter designs a door and makes it. In this way, he turns matter into effect; he is the cause over matter by shaping it into objects. However, one now easily comes under attack. God forbid if one makes a mistake and the door is not satisfactory. Hence, the manufacturer is responsible for his product. This is another reason why production is given a bad name. One could make a mistake and be chided for it. Some forget that if nothing is produced, one has nothing for personal use. It is better if someone makes a few mistakes every now and then than to have a world of naggers and inept* individuals who achieve absolutely nothing at all!

Too often one is turned into an effect through the possession of matter, whereby matter determines one's existence. You have to take care of its preservation, otherwise it will fall into disrepair. Freedom now means the ability to let go of it so that one can say that someone can be free when he is the cause. Cause is a piece of ability.

The majority of the human race now demands to be an effect. One goes to the theater, invites one to a leisurely visit to a restaurant to eat, rides the roller coaster, or enjoys other people's ideas from a book. However, nothing is created out of the effect itself. Only being an effect results in inability and a slave existence because only one's own ideas and actions will change something.

Now what is more important in life … causing things or being the effect of something? Well, pleasure is an effect, and providing a service is a cause. Of course, one can enjoy one's own performance because the joy of it is the effect. Thus, there should be a healthy relationship between cause and effect.

Since one as spirit is cause over matter and life, one also should be cause over death. There is no ultimate thing like death. The spirit cannot help but live; however, there will come a time in which the body has become useless and only causes pain.

So it is in life that the desire for joyful experience also invites pain, and you have no choice but to experience both. Not having experienced all of this means not having lived, and maybe you are clever enough to avoid the negative.

Remember: Possessions only come in a package with good and bad sides and the pleasant and the unpleasant. It always requires your time because the more one has, the more time it will require. Carpe diem*? Seize the day and don't spoil it with negative thoughts.

Relationship and Logic

Yes, what does one have to do with the other? How does logic fit into a relationship or a relationship into logic? A relationship is basically a kind of connection between two beings. These two beings now use communication as a means of understanding. If one breaks down the word communication, one finds the Latin word *communis*, which means something like common. Communication, therefore, is something that one has in common, a form of reality, something with which there is agreement.

Everyone in life now has personal views on how things should be. If someone has the same point of view and has the same ideas, then you can get along with him very well because you both are on the same wavelength.

Have you ever watched an old couple? They often do not have much to say to one another even though they live side by side. What has happened? One thing is that one is significantly more stupid than the other one. He cannot understand things as well, and he cannot recognize what one thing has to do with the other or how one thing affects the other. The more intelligent of the two now tries to explain something to the other. Well, the stupid one just does not understand it, even after it was explained for the fifth time. So, what is going on now? Each will likely start to get angry with the other. Subsequently, the clever one may say to the other that he is too stupid for that and the dim one will now be huffy*.

Now play this game day after day and year after year. At some point, the smarter one thinks that there is no value in explaining something to the other or even in communicating with the other.

This is likewise true with performing various rituals, like keeping order, taking care of affairs, dealing with other people, and so on. Since one has his own idea of how matters are to be dealt with, and the other, of course, has his own rituals, it can become an interpersonal crisis with one of them walking away and shaking his head in disbelief.

Now, the more one shows a comprehensible, logical behavior, the more one can assume that the other agrees with one's behavior. Not agreeing means "to divide," which results in a discrepancy*. The more discrepancies one has, the more the relationship goes down the drain until it runs dry, and one can no longer speak of a relationship – no more reference!

In this sense, logic, common education, and knowledge require utmost attention. Hence, there should also be lively communication between one another to share and understand the ideas that the other has. At the beginning of the relationship, being in love may be a strong magnet; however, over time, a lack of understanding develops, which is simply due to insufficient logic and too little common knowledge, which results in reversing the polarity of the magnet and one repelling each another.

So when choosing a partner, one should make sure that one has an intellectual counterpart as a partner, either equally stupid or equally intelligent. Establishing this as a foundation enables a level of consent. The common themes that life brings with it are held at the level of the intellect, either very deep or quite shallow. Getting someone to be a deep diver when he just learned to swim just does not work!

What Makes the Human Complicated?

What makes the human complicated? It is his "logic!" He confuses logic with stimulus reaction. For the sake of illustration, one could divide thinking into three categories:

1. Identified thinking (thinking in terms of equation; stimulus reaction)
2. Associative thinking (thinking by connecting things together)

3. Differentiated thinking (thinking by differentiating things from one another)

Take for example a political party prior to the federal election, which has construction or expansion of Autobahnen (highways) as a program for the improvement of Germany. Some will now speak out indignantly* and revolt, "What Autobahnen? Hitler* already build Autobahnen, and these only served one purpose!" Or as an acquaintance of mine told a coworker, "Work makes (you) free!" The coworker was shocked and told him that this sentence could be found above the entrance gates of the former Nazi concentration camps. What form of thinking do we have here? It is identified as associative thinking. What does Hitler have to do with Autobahnen in today's life?

The person who links Hitler and his intentions to the building of Autobahnen in today's life, lives with much of his mind in the past and is not really in the present. This person is paranoid, psychotic, loopy and mentally ill!

How many chances do you think a brilliant politician, full of idealism and committed to the good of a people, would have if he ran for a country as head of government under the name of Adolf Hitler? This name is so energetically charged and connected with the atrocities of an almost all-destroying Second World War that the human starts to freak out just by hearing this name.

Autobahnen? Differentiated thinking? Well, what is the purpose of society with its intentions, structures, and connections to neighboring countries? – Autobahnen! And if someone wants to tell you something about war again, then he has too much Adolf Hitler on his mind.

But this form of mental illness in the form of logic can be found right in one's own surroundings. One says, "Your ex has a new partner. She is an entrepreneur and works from home. Yes, your ex needs someone with a strong hand." An angry reply follows, "What is that supposed to mean now? Am I stupid, and do I not stand firmly with both of my legs in life?"

Thus, one "wrong" word results in the greatest war in the house. Unintentionally, or not, one pushes a person's button, and he goes crazy. But it is not only the words that trigger these reactions. Smell, clothing, behavior or just the appearance of the other are enough to activate the energetically charged events. For example, one sees the other for the first time and does not like him! Or one sees him for the first time and falls in love with him!

Now, what does the person dislike, or what does he love? Is it the person in front of him or a similar experience from the past? Of course, thinking means using past perceptions and coping with the tasks and problems of the present and the future. But it does not mean that past bad experiences keep repeating themselves. That would be thinking in equations. A thought includes association, identification and differentiation.

One wants to unscrew a bolt. From past experience, one knows that a wrench is needed to do this (association). At the same moment, one realizes that it is a size 10 spanner wrench that will fit (identification). However, the current situation involves a different bolt, a different environment and a different tool (differentiation).

Just because one had poor quality tools in the past and, as a result, messed up the work, does not mean that one is again messing up current similar work. One can recognize and change the factors in the now. The factors from the past are not the factors in the present. I mean, some no longer pick up a wrench because they have hurt themselves with it in the past (identification).

If you go to the psychologist with a problem, and he asks what kind of problem you had as a child with your mother's or father's sexual organ, then he is trying to address a previous problem to solve a current problem. Soberly realize that the treatment will fail from the above approach. Every human has his own specific experiences, and only one's own mind will be able to solve one's own problem. The therapist only needs to ask the right questions. Psychology and associative thinking? The favorite game of a modern and confused society. I mean, a cigar is a cigar and not a phallic symbol* ... Rorschach*!

The psychologist or psychiatrist always has tried to solve human madness with some form of logic based on some theory. That does not work ... which has been proven thus far. One does not solve madness with logic, no more than a little madness could defeat madness! One only has to discover the force that feeds the madness, and once one eliminates the force, the madness also stops!

What messes up the human's differentiated thinking? It is not the conscious experiences once made. that impose themselves upon the human, or the accidents that he sees, the quarrels that he had, and the mishaps or frauds that have happened to him. It is the events that affect him with such force that he was knocked out and became unconscious, like birth! These events form the hidden influence that can be reactivated at the push of a button, and the human cannot access them from his memory because they are blocked off by the walls of pain and unconsciousness. Regarding birth ... every human being has had one. I think that it has become clear by now that information cannot be stored in cells. The cell is only a manifestation of energy, whereby this energy needs information in order to be able to work specifically.

Look, you usually make a mistake only once. If the soup is too salty, you will use less salt the next time. If the screw is too weak to hold the item, you will use a larger one next time or one made of a different material. And if you experience rejection from your fellow human beings through your behavior, you will change your behavior. You analyze the source of the error so that it does not happen to you again the next time.

However, you will not be able to do that with the experiences that lie behind the curtain of oblivion ... for they are closed off! As a result, these locked-off experiences always push a certain behavior on the person, and the person seems unable to change, causing him to make the same mistake over and over again! It is like the husband of an acquaintance of mine who hit his son with a leather belt; the husband cries bitterly in the evening because of his behavior. Despite good persuasion and confessions of improvement, the husband could not desist* and hit his son again and again.

Logic. Consistency? From what experiences does the person bend the expected result? The "logic" of the human being has gone so far astray that he is led by insane explanations to voluntary ingest toxins and waste materials. For "therapeutic" purposes, one drinks his own urine and swallows snake venom (medication)! Thus, a dissociation* takes place; there are no longer any connections. Things are no longer associated with one another on the basis of natural laws, and the human still believes that he is normal!

Hence, the human lives in a lie eaten up by prejudices and tries to unite the present with the past. Only death seems to be able to free him from this curse.

Mature for a Relationship

Well, when is one ready for a relationship? If one looks into one's circle of acquaintances, one will notice that relationships are constantly falling apart, be they marriages or partnerships. Were the partners mature enough for a relationship? I mean, the ship ran aground, and it does not go any further.

What is a 2D*? Let us disassemble a relationship into its component parts. There are two people and a common intention: The experience of love is the essential foundation. A human consists of spirit, soul, body and mind.

The soul as a subordinate entity* solely follows the task of taking care of the body. It sends the sensation to force the maintenance of bodies, like the feeling of hunger and the sensations around sexuality, such as love, hate, jealousy, and so forth. Every kind of life, be it animal, plant or human, inevitably has a soul; it contains a complete set of data for the formation of an organism. It is immaterial and cannot die. Plants also have these sensations – they even react to music.

The body, which consists of individual cells that also live, sends impulses such as pain, warmth, cold, and so on. Each of these sensations is sent with a certain intensity. For example, one can be very hungry or not very hungry. The strength of the intensity results in the urgency. Pain can represent the greatest force because it indicates an impending loss. Severe pain is something that the person reacts to quite quickly.

The mind is the information filing system of the human being. There, made perceptions are stored. The perceptions are charged differently, contain more or less emotion (energy) and affect the urgency. For example, when you are at home, and it smells like the time your hair dryer was burning, then you will immediately check to see what is going on.

The spirit, meaning the person himself, is the boss of the store. It evaluates the information from the soul, mind and body and determines what to do and what not to do. The spirit is also immaterial and immortal. In contrast to the animal and plant world, usually only the human being has a spirit, which does not mean that if the person absolutely wants, he also can be something else, maybe a worm, an elephant or a flower. The above brief explanation of spirit, soul, mind and body should serve as a guide to ultimately determine what belongs where.

When is something mature for a relationship? It is most obviously seen on the body. The body has passed through puberty, and the soul now gives the full impulse to preserve the species – love and sexuality. Thus, the body would be mature for a relationship or, to put it more precisely, for reproduction. In the animal kingdom, the whole matter is quite straightforward. One mates and goes one's own way or stays together until the offspring are fully fledged and can fend for themselves. Many species even stay together for life.

What does it mean when the partner says, "I love you"? It means that he receives an impulse from the soul and interprets this impulse as a feeling of love. This feeling "fuses*" the sexes together on a physical level, and when one separates and still is in love, it just hurts terribly because the soul has its precautions. So, the person plays this love-body game because of the impulses that he receives from the soul to play this game.

Can a person be mature for a relationship? How do relationships work with humans? One sees the other, finds him interesting, exchanges a few words, falls in love and has sex. However, in our civilized world, this comes with a lot of responsibility, including children and a lot of money that are part of marriage. Thus, it takes a certain intellect to support this unit called family in a civilization.

One is mature for a relationship when one has inner values like loyalty, reliability, empathy, a good portion of selflessness, understanding, insight, responsibility, decision-making power, cooperation and inner strength because one should be a friend to one's partner and be for him and not against him! It is of no use to run after the impulse of the soul; this impulse alone does not keep a relationship together. In the end, it is the person himself with his attitude who is decisive for the existence of a relationship!

The person himself as a spiritual being is free. With a body, he has actually given up all freedom, and with every additional dynamic, he loses a bit more freedom. A child as a human being has the most freedom. He is fed, receives clothing and accommodation and does not have to worry about anything. Then, over the course of time with the inevitable assumption of responsibility and the obligation to take care of things, freedom gradually decreases. But the fact is that freedom itself does not cause happiness; the human is happy when he has something!

As a result, when the person enters into a relationship, he will have a big problem. And that is he will no longer be able to pursue his own interests to the extent that he does now because he has a new part of his life that requires time and attention. There are two beings who share their time with one another and two thought households that should be connected to one. It is a difficult matter because it requires lively communication. How else will the other determine what to do and what not to do?

Some already have a "steady" relationship in their youth with so many of them spending their time on the couch holding hands. Youth is actually the most beautiful and exciting time in a person's life. One is free and unburdened by heavy thoughts, which only come through later experiences. Usually, one still lives at home and does not have to worry about one's own livelihood. One walks through life without the heavy burden of responsibility.

As the person gets older, very often the relationship falls apart because one does not know how to behave in a relationship, and one does not know oneself, much less the other. One hears some talk about having missed out on life because of the relationship, and some even try to catch up on everything. Think back ... how were things in your first relationship? How often were you restricted and not allowed to do what you wanted to do? How did you feel afterwards? Once an acquaintance said to me, "Tonight I am going to paint the town red*, but without a shadow!" Well, the shadow was his girlfriend, and, whenever she was around, he just could not behave the way he would have liked. A relationship takes freedom!

This means to experience the things that one would like to experience. However, when one has experienced all things, one knows how they are, and one does not necessarily have to experience them anymore. The person languishes* in his thoughts and is satisfied to put the thought aside only when he has experienced it. Therefore, when one is young, one should really kick up one's heels so that later on, one does not have the need to catch up on everything.

Of course, it is difficult to combine a relationship with freedom to give the other free space, especially at a young age, because one is afraid of losing the other. Likewise, this feeling of having to be with the other is very strong, and it hurts to be apart. On occasion, the partner should insist that the other also go out alone with his friends, and the partner should understand why. By the same token, the evening also can be spoiled when the other is not there because one longs for him. Here it is important to reevaluate.

Speaking of youth and kicking up one's heals. This is important so that later you do not feel like you have missed it all and blame your significant other – at least you did it!

Mature for a relationship? How much of yourself do you give up to allow the other to have a "friendly playing field" while remaining with you? To what extent are you ready to shift your values parameters? Remember, do not shift too much. Otherwise, you will no longer live your life, and you will become unhappy. As a result, the relationship will become unhappy and fail. Listening to music that one does not want to hear or driving somewhere one does not enjoy can be put away from time to time.

Victim

This is what my mentor says in the axioms*: **"The greatest goal in this universe is the creation of an effect"** (LRH).

Yes, one can roughly divide this effect into two directions: positive and negative. Positive, for example, would be admiration for a prize in sports, good looks or constructive projects. Of course, anything related to destruction would be negative.

A victim is someone to whom something has happened. The human plays this game quite superbly, "Look what happened to me!" What does he intend to achieve with it? Attention, of course! To the extent that he receives attention, he achieves an effect. Some seem unable to live without attention.

Recently, I heard on the radio that children's skin allergies improve when they are separated by their parents. Even though the medic does not understand the mechanism behind the matter, he has observed this case well. Humans actually present an illness to get attention. This reminds me of my grandmother. My brother, who lived in her house at the time, told her that he wanted to move in with his girlfriend. Lo and behold, my grandmother got a rheumatic attack because her dearest grandson wanted to leave.

It often can be observed in children that they are completely psyched* when visitors arrive. All sorts of stuff are dragged in or the visitor is pulled through the house. And they all only want one thing: to find confirmation that they exist. If you hug and cuddle the child a little, all seems to be good, and she goes on her way. However, some adults seem to have very high deficits. Just watch the talk shows on television and look at the provocative brand clothing, tattoos and piercings. One thing I realized was the more the person played the victim role, the more he is incapable.

Being a victim in itself indicates that something has happened to one, that one was not fully focused at a certain point in time, or that one was just acting foolish – except maybe for those who just could not help it. Another possibility is that one has made some other stupid mistake and Karma* caught up with him. In any case, one is never completely innocent. The victim just lacks insight and the ability to relate things to one another to recognize in advance what will harm one. In this sense, a victim displays a certain stubbornness because he is unable to let go of the thought that dictates his behavior and to replace it with a new thought.

You have become a victim yourself when you are with someone who is obviously "always" a victim. He cannot get his stuff done and drags all sorts of problems to you because he cannot get them resolved. In addition, money disappears, the mail does not find the direct way to the mailbox, and when one includes the victim into one's prayers, it collapses like a house of cards. These people are very emotionally sensitive and fragile due to their own misdeeds!

Should you ask a favor, he dramatizes about how difficult everything is and all that he has to do. Furthermore, he will not be frugal* with bad criticism. In life it is not easy to get along with people like that.

Have you become a victim's victim? He is the vampire who sucks out your life force, and you do not get anything back. All that remains is a bunch of broken shards*! Also, be careful with the "interesting" ones in this world, they can be a danger to you.

Family

So here you are, the basis of all life that forms matter into an organism and holds it together. I am referring to you yourself not the body, but a spiritual being, a thetan*.

Now what is this game called family? I mean, this is wonderful. One has found one another, is in love, wears rose-colored glasses, wants to move in together and get married. One enjoys the other's company and is happy to be together. At least one is in love, and that brings happiness. Love is an interesting matter; nobody knows exactly how it works or its origin. One just has this feeling, and it is this sensation that "fuses" one together.

Living together as man and woman is an endeavor*. A thetan has grabbed himself a male body, the other a female one, and both are playing the body game. Both have their own goals and intentions and their own preferences. One likes eggs for breakfast, and the other does not like the smell of eggs with Maggi* at all. The woman wants to go on vacation to the Riviera, and the man prefers to climb around the mountains. The cabinet should be functional, but the woman believes that it is not nice and does not quite match the other furniture. The man enjoys watching James Bond while the woman enjoys watching *Sex and the City*.

Thus, one has one's daily small war and is forced to make compromises in one way or another. The male body is different from the female one, and both are different in terms of performance. Usually the man can lift more iron and run faster than the woman should the idea of doing sports together arise to bring some competition into the matter. Hence, there are also different interests that everyone should be able to pursue in their own form.

The only thing that connects man and woman physically is sexuality, which both can indeed do with each other. After all, that is why man and woman actually exist. So, what can one really do with one another without being dependent on the body's specifications? Examples include mental things, such as watching something together and chatting about it, or planning projects and bringing them to life.

As far as the generation of thoughts are concerned, both have the same prerequisites, and both can develop these images called ideas. The whole life is a dynamic project, and whichever idea is best should be pursued because it is obvious that, due to myopia* and mistakes, nobody has come far. The man in the house may have a problem if the woman has better ideas, but, often enough, one can see that the woman of the house is in charge. Nevertheless, one should be aware that two spiritual beings have joined forces to walk through life, both of which deserve equal respect as beings.

At some point, the topic of children comes up. After all what is a family without children? Once the little screamer has seen the light of day, the family game is played together. Nonetheless, the child is a thetan, a thetan in a small body with its goals, intentions and preferences, even though not yet as obvious. The human may say that life is a coming and going, but it is just a being. You are actually not going anywhere – only to the next maternity ward where you grab a new body and "forget" the past. I mean, somehow you got into this one.

I am not talking nonsense here. The people who have been in a sufficient number of sessions in a regression look at their past, and all tell the same thing: old body, new body, old body, new body, and so on. You can believe it or not; that does not change the fact that water flows downhill.

One of the main reasons why the human's behavior is exalted* in regard to children is because children have children again, and you can start over when the old body passes the temporal. Your children are your future, and who does not want it to continue somehow to come full circle? In fact, life itself is a narrowing spiral. From body to body, the human's health deteriorates, and his mental ability decreases.

Incidentally, the word family originates from Latin *famulus*, which means something like helper or servant. Who is helping whom and how? Woman and man are independent beings. They can go through life on their own, although it can be easier together without making it difficult interpersonally. Many see the meaning of life in the family to be there for the other, to help one another and to give consolation when the mood is in the basement. This is how one helps each other.

Often, one can hear the parents of children say that all they do is for their children. Well, what does one owe to children? These children have their goals, intentions, and, when the day comes, they will go their own way. As *Der Große Konz*[5] said, "The capital that one has saved should be depleted when one dies." However, on a personal note, one never really knows when that is. A good education is all that one owes one's children.

Here I would like to start by saying that I have exhausted the subject of training* in detail: There is no good training. Feeding the child, dressing him warmly and sending him to school is not enough. One must teach the children how to help themselves in life, to defend themselves and to have a good idea of what is important in life. This is the service that parents should render to the family: Guide the child in how to respond to life's events – a real help! In the same way, the state should help its citizens because we are all one big family.

Marriage (= German *Heirat:* home + advice)? Who would have thought that? Every word has a deeper meaning, which actually should be a guide for behavior – the word and the function that results from the meaning. One set up camp somewhere to advise one another! And because one should actually be together for a lifetime, one should advise one another over the whole life, regarding activities in which to engage and solving the problems that arise from them.

Wedlock? This word comes from the Old English *wedlāc,* marriage bond, from wedd pledge + -*lāc,* suffix denoting activity. It is the will of life itself that binds forever and wants to live forever.

A Place in the Heart of the Other

What does it mean to have a place in the heart of the other? Well, the heart does not store any information. You have a "place in the heart" of the other when the other's mind revolves around you.

You cannot force your place into the other person's heart! If you act too strongly, or are too pushy, he will withdraw. On the other hand, if you do not seek contact and do not draw attention to yourself, the other will think that he is indifferent to you and that you are not interested.

Yes, a difficult matter! Not to be intrusive on the one hand and to show interest on the other. You will find out by the other person's reaction. Is he annoyed*? Is the other person's mood kind to you? Does he keep in touch?

Something can be done so that the other includes you in his heart, and something has to be done that this place is preserved when it was given to you. What does the other think about when he thinks of you? Does he think about what you did to him, whether you were or will be his friend, a good time, a time full of complications, a heap of problems or suffering and anger?

He will think about whether he really wants to have something to do with you and whether he really enjoys your company. Quite simply, he will consider which side the scale leans toward: Is there more joy or more discomfort?

When the other seeks contact with you, he lets you understand that you mean something, that you represent a value to him and that there is something that he wants to have.

Also, do not gift the other a lot of material things because he will only like you for these. Instead, give him what only life itself can give: attention, understanding, warmth, love and tenderness. Be a friend to the other! After all, the other should love you as a person and not your material gifts.

The Relationship Fails

There are some who believe that a relationship runs automatically. You will then have a beautiful house and a beautiful garden when you take care that it is in order. This universe is a living universe in which things change, evolve and interact. It is the same with a relationship. One changes and evolves, is affected by the environment and has to take care of a relationship so that it is in order. One has to nurture and maintain it and actively deal with it. An engine also runs automatically but only when fuel is added, and its oil and water levels are occasionally checked. Just like the engine needs energy to function, a relationship needs energy to exist. One has to put something into this relationship.

A relationship is not just the physical attraction that boils down to sexuality. Above all, it is an alliance between two beings in which the alliance is based on various rules, expressed or not. Compliance with the rules guarantees the existence of this alliance. By violating them too often, the relationship breaks up. You will find that the following codex sets out the foundations for an alliance.

Is a relationship a relationship when one has sex with each other? Sex is only the bonus that deepens the feeling of one another. A relationship that only exists through sex is not a relationship between two beings. It is a relationship between two bodies that breaks when one has more desire for another body and feels more pleasure there.

Some recognize "love" by the tingling sensation in the stomach – the first step to a crash landing! Of course, a relationship requires mutual attractiveness and the lust for each other, but not understanding each other will break the relationship in a short time or in the long term. So far, in establishing a relationship, the sexual impulse has been the only measure of the human to recognize his "love." That is why he constantly gets disappointed!

There is a reason why one no longer gets along so well with the other, and the desire for the other has fallen asleep. Of course, the simplest reason would be to say that one no longer wants to continue. This does not need to be further justified, but it can also be that there are other reasons.

It is always a matter of communication to find out what is going on; however, both should be ready to communicate and so be able to talk with the other without giving free rein to one's emotions. Communication should be a sober and matter-of-fact conversation with clear representations.

A relationship between the sexes is clearly shown by space. Love was defined as: "The desire to occupy the same space as the other." Contrarily, hate is characterized by distance. Whether the other person loves you is shown simply by the distance he keeps from you and whether he tries to be close to you. When someone wants to spend time with you and feels well understood and respected, then he certainly has a relationship with you!

What did I write previously? The secret is the separation. Have you ever stolen something small in a store as a child? How did you feel when you got to the checkout? Would you not have liked to steer clear of the cashier? At least you had a feeling of doing this, a feeling to keep a lot of distance. This feeling arose because you did something that was wrong and that violated the covenant* of coexistence.

As in a relationship, when one breaks the covenant, love extinguishes, as well as the feeling of being together, and one keeps one's distance. Interestingly enough, by fully acknowledging one's violations, the urge to have space dissolves. One can stumble from one relationship to the next and shipwreck there again only because one does not reveal one's violations that he has made. As a partner, one should recognize when the other wants to give up because the current fate will likely show itself over and over again. Yes, of course, it is easier to run away rather than to confront the problem; however, you will always run away from yourself ... from your own thoughts!

Many partners cite the reason for separation is that they no longer want to hurt the other. Well, by revealing one's secret violations of the covenant of togetherness, one no longer has the impulse to separate. Entering into a relationship means entering into a contract whether the terms of the contract are known or not because everyone has a certain idea of what not to do in a relationship!

Frequently criticizing and complaining about the other person means that one is different and that one is distancing oneself. One also distances oneself when he gets hurt by the other, be it through violence or bad words, which brings us back to the definition of friend: The one who does not do this.

Accusing the other of all that he has done? Well, what have you done? That is how it is; however, by knowing how the human being functions, one can get along with him. A relationship fails not only because of what one has done but also because one should have done something about it. So, it is also up to the other to say what to do. And do not wait for the barrel to overflow ... note when it fills!

Consider: When someone reports his misconduct, he does so to save the relationship by trying to be honest and sincere. If the deed was probably not that of a "friend," the exposing of such is an effort to continue to be "friendly." Therefore, you should accept the confession as an effort to maintain the friendship, even if it is difficult to digest. So, consider your reaction, and maybe it is even better to sleep one night over a decision.

Thus, from the very beginning, the human cut his own throat by breaking covenants through dishonesty and insincerity, be it with his employer or the rest of the world. He executes himself through illness and inability so that he can no longer do bad deeds.

What are the reasons for making the decision to go one's separate ways? First and foremost, one is unhappy. What are the things that make for a happy relationship?

Entering into a relationship with someone has a goal. One is not happy by not achieving this goal or when there are circumstances that stand in the way or have a serious effect on the goal. One could say that the primary goal of a relationship is to experience love. One wants to have someone to love and wants the other person's love in return. At least that is what the individual imagines under the term love, like security, affection, not being alone, sexuality, having a place where one belongs, familiarity, understanding, communication and problem solving, ultimately everything that one experiences in life with a relationship.

No longer a real relationship? It is the common goals and the common undertakings that strengthen a relationship and give it a foundation and reason for movement.

Irreconcilable* differences? How much is one able to think another thought? How much is one able to understand the other and move away from one's own point of view?

The impulse of affection is the real reason to get closer. To really get to know one another, one must know the other person's inclination, peculiarities, preferences, reactions, and so on. This is a process that takes time. A long-term relationship that should be harmonious means that one coordinates all of this, which has a lot to do with compromise and tolerance. After all, there are two beings with their own ideas, and it is often not so easy to make one out of two ideas.

An acquaintance of mine who married for the second time was of the opinion that one should not get married until one is 30 years old quite simply because one possesses more reason at that age, and one is more aware of the things in life that are important. Being in love is a nice thing, but it is something completely different to live a life with one's partner and always have him around. There is a bit more than just being in love, like running a household, keeping order, planning and solving the tasks and problems that arise each day. This results in a daily routine; it takes time to reconcile family and professional life because there are only 24 hours in a day, and there also should be an end of the workday!

A wife would not want a man who has high support obligations from a previous relationship and, for this reason alone, can no longer take care of himself, only bringing a lot more problems with him because everything should somehow work in the end.

A household with children is a 24-hour job without a weekend when one could sleep in properly. The reward is an inner feeling of doing the right thing. One is there for the other, and one is motivated because of this assumed obligation. To just let oneself go is not an option.

If this job were messed up, the whole world would actually be messed up because without this basic social building block called family, nothing would function.

Quite fundamentally, the word friend provides sufficient guidelines on how one is to behave in a relationship. Someone who is not a friend does things that does not please one – it's just that easy! Consequently, the behavior towards one another plays a big role.

Every game is based on very specific rules. By breaking these rules, one loses the game. An overriding rule in a relationship is the thematic* devaluation. Devaluation means that the person's worth has diminished. Everyone has his own individual worth; one can do this better and the other that.

Devaluation in itself counts particularly in the respect that every individual has regardless of their skills. It is the dignity of the person. To say, "You are stupid" to someone gives the other side the impulse to defend himself, and it is very easy for one word to result in another. Soon the pot boils over.

Of course, it takes self-discipline to pull oneself together and not to rumble into one's own emotional outburst. In fact, all too often it is the case that one hurts the ones the most whom he loves the most. How else would it work? Because if one does not have an emotional bond to the other, one will not be hurt much by him!

Devaluing does not only mean not appreciating the person, but also the things that he does, denigrating* the things with which the person himself identifies. Devaluation is also ignorance. One ignores things that have no value. There is also a devaluation, even if indirectly, when one does not respond to the wishes of the partner within the relationship – of course, wishes also have their tolerance limits. Why should one love someone who does not appreciate him?

However, the person himself plays a big role. One could say that the relationship is as stable as each individual within the relationship. After all, the person exists first of all as an individual. If the person loses himself, then he will also lose the relationship. There is no point in giving up on oneself with all of one's goals, intentions and inclinations. When one gives up on oneself, he becomes unhappy with himself. One should ensure one's own happiness and then align one's goals and intentions for the relationship with one's own goals and intentions. By not doing this, not only does he perish, but so does the relationship and the partner.

Therefore, make sure that your partner still has room to breathe in the relationship!

Still a Few More Trifles

When everyday life has returned: Do not get angry with your partner and do not reproach* him. Have you ever stood in front of someone who was really angry with you? How did you feel? Well, you got his emotion, and it intimidated you. When you meet your partner again, you will be careful not to make him angry, and you will be careful what you say to him. You also will try not to do what made the other angry.

Thus, the emotion of the other influences your behavior, and you become less and less yourself. And the less you are yourself, the more unhappy you will become. The fear of expressing a mishap or a wish to the other becomes too great, so one begins to lie. This means the real end of the relationship when one can no longer be honest with the other.

This is similar to when one reminds the other of what one helped him with or what he is always doing wrong. You are forcing the person to suffer his own consequences, to stop asking you or to handle things completely on his own. This is a step towards the end of the partnership because one starts to handle things himself and no longer wants to talk about it.

Of course, one does not always have time or the patience for the other, but one can still pull oneself together and show a certain amount of understanding simply for the sake of the partnership!

Force yourself to be friendly to people around you, even if they are not. Do not give unkindness a chance to spread further. Instead, work on making this world a friendly one because it brings you back joy. One hears mothers say that there is nothing comparable to what a child can give. It is the joy that the child radiates that touches one, and one can feel the power of the emotional wave lengths.

One cannot exist with or without the other? Yes, of course. When there are no basics about how to get along with the other, constant quarreling will result.

My women's stories? Maybe it is enough to say that they cost me a lot of time, nerves and money, all on the debit side of the balance sheet. What did I have? I was allowed to experience what affection, hope, longing, warmth and tenderness mean. I was allowed to experience what love is all about - the whole package - in good times and in bad. And you know what? It is a part of life; it adds some excitement to the matter and does not make life so boring. It is entertainment, a game.

The partner left me after I helped. Oh well. I know that it made her feel better, and it will probably happen that I also will be helped when I am really in a bind. I can thank the person now for being there! And this person probably only exists because someone has already helped him when he was in a tight spot!

And yes, women seem to get more and more complicated with increasing age. No wonder, too many bad experiences! Women will probably say the same about men. The good thing about experience is that you know exactly what you do not want!

If a person reacts quite violently to a matter, he himself is not innocent in this regard.

Resolve inconsistencies immediately. The barrel fills up slowly and is often emptied with a big bang.

Take responsibility with your partner. Keep this in mind and help to make things work. Arguing brings loneliness. Work together to face everyday life. See also the second dynamic codex at the end of this text.

"A plant will grow and thrive as long as one creates the habitat in which it is possible – <u>and this requires constant doing!</u>"

Grant each other time and hobbies without infringing on the area of the other one. There are eight dynamics!!!

Should incidents arise that affect you both, such as the visit of parents or a friend, talk it over first so that the two of you make it possible by mutual consent. Do not take the initiative and invite someone without your partner's knowledge; this will only lead to vexation*.

In the case of a household with both working full time, open a "house-account" at the bank into which everyone deposits the same amount per month. From this account, the direct maintenance costs, such as rent, utilities and groceries, are paid. Should one of you be a special connoisseur, then he pays this extra himself.

You determine the monthly costs with a household account book as "evidence." It must be managed in such a way that the individual for whom the item is intended is clearly identified. For example, my household account book contains the following breakdown: food, cleaning supplies, house expenses, purchases "house," car, common costs with each line item linked to the one for whom it is intended, i.e., Kerstin, Wolfgang, cat.

Do not allow the partner to always invite you because he will hold it against you at some point. Be there for one another and help each other, but if you take, you must also give.

Make a note of the joint purchases and keep the receipts. In the event of a separation, one person will take the purchase with him, and the other will receive money or something else in return. Sit down together and settle it fairly because you will never know how and if you will meet again. An unfair division brings resentment!

One always meets twice in life!

"Never try to upset your fellow human beings around you!" Remember you have been friends and know each other. A broken relationship does not mean that friends can no longer be there for each other.

A family and children make everything more difficult. But bear in mind when you find yourself dying in this relationship, your surroundings will perish as well. Therefore, draw a line and begin a new and happy existence.

The important thing in life is never to give up! Remember that you have legs. If you ever fell at some point, you can get up again, and if you do not succeed in this life, then you will succeed in the next. You just cannot give up!!!

Perseverance is the most important thing that one can have. One could place it above intelligence. Intelligence may make a lot of things easier, but only with perseverance will you achieve your goal.

Always keep your eyes and ears open. When things are complicated, then there are probably people in the background who do not want things to be really understood. They probably do not know about it themselves.

The world and its essence* are simple. When someone has really understood something, he can easily explain it to you. You just have to pay attention to understand all of the words, as already described in detail in my texts.

Something else: **Never forget your friends. Never!!! You never know when you will need them.**

In addition, one has a precise way to free oneself from the shackles of the mind and, therefore, is able to think straight out accident-free. There is functional knowledge there for every aspect of life, be it understanding, learning, communication, discovering and increasing personal skills, psychosomatic illnesses, beginning, running and maintaining a marriage, raising children, getting along with others, solving drug problems, detox programs, decriminalization in society, management, financial management, administration, public relation, ethics, recognizing and crushing oppression, and so on.

A word about psychosomatic illnesses. Definition: From Greek, *psyche* = soul + *soma* = body. Actually, it refers to how the mind with energy affects the body and changes its shape. For example, when you hit your finger, you feel pain in the form of electrical energy. More pain, more energy that is sent out by the cell and perceived by you. This energy, as well as the deformed finger, are stored as experience (facsimile = mental image picture with measurable energy). If one now perceives sounds or smells or sees something similar to a previous experience, the energy flows out of this facsimile and, with pain, changes the body structure to warn you of a "danger point." This produces a corresponding behavior of the person with the disadvantage that one is "sick." However, this is for the "protection" of the body. This contains about 80% of the known disease catalog, like migraines, stomach ulcers, arthritis, cancer, and so on, as well as susceptibility to viruses and bacteria. It also includes all neuroses and psychoses, for these are the forms of behavior that dictate the energy from the person's facsimile – a forced behavior!

Note: This knowledge was written purely out of observation and is not simply the opinion of a human. The human needs knowledge that he can rely on, as well as stable data that will help him go through life and help him get up again when he falls. He will have knowledge only through clarity. The human will only be able to go through life as successfully as things are really clear. After all, accidents often happen in the fog!

Right and Wrong

Let us now turn to a very philosophical topic: right and wrong. By that I mean, when is right right and wrong wrong?

Well, let us see what I make of it with my limited mental horizon. As always, I try to keep this topic very brief so as not to strain the reader with longwinded representations. Let us keep the whole matter short and sweet and limit ourselves to the basics. As the saying goes: Brevity is the source of wit.

As already mentioned before there is a scale to everything, from completely wrong to completely right. As it is with this topic, right and wrong are usually situational.

An acquaintance of mine went to a shaman, and the subject of right and wrong came up. The shaman said that his alignment would stand between right and wrong, i.e., being neutral. The acquaintance should have asked him the following questions: What should I do if I am on a tour of a lake on a passenger ship, and a child falls overboard in the middle of the lake? Should I go to the captain and tell him to go on under any circumstances or stop the ship to save the child? What if I didn't do anything, like being neutral? Would I be good or bad then? With the example above, I want to express that right and wrong take part in the real world. People like to generalize and lose reference to reality.

There is nothing worse than stubborn rules or commandments. For example: Thou shalt not kill. However, by going to war for your country, this commandment is suddenly invalid. You would even be punished if you did not do it!

Let us take a look at a few basic parameters* by which one can measure right and wrong. Here again is the definition of reason: "The doing or refraining of actions that will bring you and your symbionts more advantages than disadvantages, now and in the future." Consider the eight dynamics*!

Problems with implementation? You do not know if what you are doing is right? Very simple:

- **Treat others as you would like to be treated yourself.**
- **Only cause things that you want to experience yourself.**

This is how you should interact with your fellow human beings, if you think that you are the victim of injustice. Ask the other: "Would you like to be treated the way you treat or have treated me?" "Would you like to receive the mess you passed on?" "It is up to you to change this; think about it!"

Every step towards happiness is a step in the right direction; every step towards unhappiness is wrong! Part of happiness is to understand yourself and the world around you - and to be able to recognize evil so that you can do something about it. Don't just turn away from evil. What if it turns to you?

Codex for the Second Dynamic

I promise
1. To make you happy.
2. To give you a feeling of security.
3. To not devalue your feelings, thoughts, opinions or behavior.
4. To maintain as much communication with you as possible, even if I have to resolve a serious resentment.
5. To help you, to stand by you and to be there for you as a partner whenever it is necessary.
6. To increase responsibility for my incorrect actions.
7. To not take pity on you but to act effectively.
8. To grant you who you are.
9. To be honest with you.
10. To not engage in sexual activities with other individuals.
11. To not force my reality on you but to act effectively and strive for understanding.
12. To not have a purely sexual relationship with you but to take care of you as a being and to form a deep bond of understanding and affection because to not understand each other and to not get along means to break the bonds of love at some point.
13. To deal with those actions that lead to an ever-higher degree of understanding and, with those actions, establish and sustain an environment in which two beings can grow and expand in this and other dynamics.

With every revealed violation of the codex by the partner, the other can point out this code, and the one who violated it is then obliged to handle the situation in a way that both are happy with the solution. Additionally, the one who violates the codex can demand that the partner helps to resolve the situation.

Your Rainbow

The wind blows the last clouds from the blue sky. The glistening light of the sun drives away the tribulation of the last raindrops.

And you see a rainbow in the blue sky. It shimmers in the most splendid colors, from an enchanting purple to a bright yellow.

You dream and think, "Will there be a pot of gold at the end of this rainbow?"

Well, you see it, this rainbow. You see it with your own eyes. It actually exists.

But there is something else:
The pot of gold!

You just have to get up and go get it!

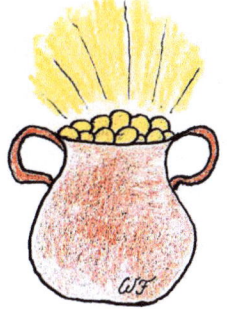

Glossary

adrenaline A hormone that is secreted by the adrenal glands, especially during times of stress.

aesthetics The teaching of the beauty of things.

affinity A spontaneous or natural liking or sympathy for someone.

amalgam filling A tooth filling with mercury content. The proportion of mercury as a heavy metal is said to have negative effects on the organism. Potential Risks: Dental amalgam contains elemental mercury. It releases low level of mercury in the form of a vapor that can be inhaled and absorbed by the lungs. High levels of mercury vapor exposure are associated with adverse effects in the brain and kidneys. However, it is problematic when fillings of different types are present, like one tooth with a gold filling and another with amalgam – the amalgam filling can dissolve.

amicable One is kind to one another and is friendly and lenient in the agreement.

anatomy [Greek *ana* = on + *tome* = to cut] The science of the construction of a body.

annoyed Feeling or showing angry irritation.

appease To pacify or placate (someone) by acceding to their demands. To relieve or satisfy (a demand or a feeling).

arm, holding up Amar Bharti has been holding up his right arm since 1973. Amar is one of the holy men of India and lives in religious asceticism*.

asceticism Severe self-discipline and avoidance of all forms of indulgence, typically for religious reasons.

authentic Real, credible. Acting in a form that one believes that it is really so, not imitated or falsified.

aversion A strong dislike or disinclination.

axiom 1. As a correctly recognized principle 2. Statement which is held to be true or correct. 3. Statement based on a law of nature.

barn thresher A threshing machine or a thresher is a piece of farm equipment that threshes grain, that is, it removes the seeds from the stalks and husks.

basta From Italian and Spanish, "Stop!" or "That's enough!"

Bravo Enlightenment magazine for people in puberty as a target group.

bastion fortification/protective barrier.

Beckham, Victoria An English singer, fashion designer and television personality.

bevy A large group of people or things of a particular kind.

blunder A stupid or careless mistake.

capital cover Financial reserves.

carpe diem [Latin "pluck the day" or "seize the day."] Phrase used by the Roman poet Horace to express the idea that one should enjoy life while one can.

celibacy [Latin *caelebs* = celibate] the professional obligation of Catholic clergymen to maintain sexual abstinence.

censorship It serves the goal in controlling the spiritual life in a religious, moral or political way.

character Actually, "features." This also includes the quirks* of the person.

coincide Occur at or during the same time.

competence The ability to do something successfully or efficiently.

complex (In psychoanalysis). An accumulation of impulses, ideas and emotions that force a behavior pattern.

communication, being in contact with Refers to the full communication cycle. It begins, changes, stops and is turned around.

covenant An agreement.

counter-thought A thought that counters or opposes another thought.

D, 2D Second dynamic, see dynamics.

decadent A decay in standards, morals, dignity, faith, and so forth.

defensive Defending; being pushed back.

dejection A sad and depressed state; low spirits.

denigrate Criticize unfairly; disparage*.

desertion Evading responsibility by fleeing. In times of war, deserters were shot.

desist Cease, abstain.

devised To plan or invent (a complex procedure, system, or mechanism) by careful thought.

dexterity A skill in performing tasks, especially with the hands.

dialectic The art of conversation.

discrepancy A lack of agreement.

disgruntled Angry or dissatisfied.

disparage Regard or represent as being of little worth.

dissociation (Actually separation). Related processes of thinking, action and behavior break down into individual uncontrolled parts and individual phenomena.

effect side The one who sees the beauty, that is, the one who is impressed by the beauty. The cause side is the source of the beauty.

eloquence Convincing mode of expression, explaining something in a convincing way, fluent or persuasive speaking or writing.

endeavor A venture or undertaking, whose success is not assured, that is quite daring in terms of its success.

entity Something that lives for itself and can exist for itself.

essence The intrinsic nature or indispensable quality of something, especially something abstract, that determines its character.

euphoria A feeling or state of intense excitement and happiness.

exploit To make full use of and derive benefit from (a resource).

exuberant Filled with or characterized by a lively energy and excitement.

facet A particular aspect or feature of something, especially of a cut gem.

farce Issue where the given intention and the given goal are no more taken seriously but ridiculed and laughed at.

fickle Changing frequently, especially in regard to one's loyalties, interests, or affection.

fidelity Faithfulness to a person, cause, or belief, demonstrated by continuing loyalty and support.

first responder Someone designated or trained to respond to an emergency such as Emergency Medical Technicians (EMTs), paramedics, firefighters and police officers.

fixed idea A thought that one has taken up and possibly pursued without having examined this thought more closely, where it leads to or what it is supposed to be.

foe An enemy or opponent.

frugal Sparing or economical with regard to money or food.

fuse Join or blend to form a single entity.

gimmick A trick or device intended to attract attention, publicity or business.

grimace An ugly, twisted expression on a person's face, typically expressing disgust, pain, or wry amusement.

hag An ugly, slatternly, or evil-looking old woman; witch.

Hamburg A major port city in northern Germany, connected to the North Sea by the Elbe River. Population as of December 30, 2019, is 1.899 million.

Hitler, Adolf Wrested Germany out of the hands of a completely incapable democracy during a time of hyperinflation and 30% unemployment. I was fortunate to talk to some people who lived during his time. My great uncle, with a glow in his eyes, told me: In the beginning, he was a total heros*! He gave bread to people who had none, gifted a stove to a family with seven children, gave people work, erected schools and cultural sites, built decent roads, and made it possible for people to walk around outside in the evening without fear because everyone knew that there was order. Unfortunately, the good he accomplished early on was undone by the evil that followed at his hands.

homo sapiens [Latin *humus* = earth + *sapiens* = wise intelligent] The modern human.

huffy Easily offended.

illicit From [Latin *illicitus*, *in-* = not + *licitus* = lawful] Usually referring to something that is not morally proper or acceptable (illicit activities).

indignantly In a manner indicating anger or annoyance at something perceived as unfair.

inept Having or showing no skill; clumsy.

infinite Limitless or endless in space, extent, or size; impossible to measure or calculate.

infinity [Latin *in-* = not + *fīnis* = boundary, limit] unlimited extent of time, space, or quantity.

intellect The ability to gain realizations and insights through thinking.

interpersonal Relating to relationships or communication between people.

intrusive Causing disruption or annoyance through being unwelcome or un-invited.

irreconcilable (Said of ideas, facts, or statements). Representing findings or points of view that are so different from each other that they cannot be made compatible.

jargon Special words or expressions that are used by a particular profession or group and are difficult for others to understand. For example, legal jargon.

Karma (In Hinduism and Buddhism). The sum of a person's actions in this and previous states of existence, viewed as deciding their fate in future existences.

Konz, Franz (1926-2013) German author and tax advisor.

languish 1. (Said of a person or other living thing). Lose or lack vitality, grow weak or feeble. 2. Suffer from being forced to remain in an unpleasant place or situation.

love, unhappily in One has fallen in love with someone one cannot have, someone who does not return love.

macho [Latin *masculus* = male, worthy of a man] Showing aggressive pride in one's masculinity. "The big macho tough guy."

madam A woman in charge of a brothel.

Maggi Also known as Maggi-Würze. Liquid seasoning, a food flavor enhancer invented in Switzerland and introduced in Germany. It is a thin concentrated dark brown liquid.

manners The way of behavior to get along with one another in a society with-out friction. Manners are part of the basic social acceptance.

monogamous [Greek, *monos* = alone + *gamein* = to marry] marriage with one partner.

marionette A puppet worked from above by strings attached to its limbs.

maxim Guiding principle.

melancholy [Greek, *melas* = black + *chole* = bile, of great dejection*] a state of mind characterized by sadness or depression.

métier [French > Old French *mistier, mestier* = divine service, function, duty, craft, profession] 1. A trade, profession, or occupation. 2. Field of activity.

mishmash A confused mixture.

morass An area of muddy or boggy ground.

myopia Nearsightedness; lack of imagination, foresight, or intellectual insight.

nib The pointed end part of a pen, which distributes the ink on the writing surface.

obtrude Become noticeable in an unwelcome or intrusive way; impose or force (something) on someone in an intrusive way.

Odyssey A quest, named after the Greek Odysseus, who came home after a long journey and many adventures.

omnipresent Present in all places at all times.

painting the town red Go out and enjoy oneself flamboyantly (idiomatic); to party or celebrate in a rowdy, wild manner, especially in a public place.

parameter [Greek *para* = beside + *metron* = measure] Characteristic quantity with the help of which statements about the structure and performance capability of something can be obtained.

phallic symbol Phallus, [Greek *phallos* = erect penis] The matter is no longer seen as a matter, but rather it is interpreted according to a complex*. For example, the construction of the tallest skyscraper is portrayed as an attention deficit and low self-esteem.

Plato An Athenian philosopher during the Classical period in Ancient Greece.

polygamy The practice or custom of having more than one wife or husband at the same time.

pornos (porn, short for pornography). The depiction of erotic behavior (as in pictures or writing) intended to cause sexual excitement.

postulate [Latin, *postulatum* = demand] A demand, a thought, an idea of how something should be.

princi [Latin *princeps* = leader > *primus* = first + *capere* = to take] This name was likely originally a nickname for someone who behaved in a regal (kingly) manner.

procreation The production of offspring, reproduction.

psyched Excited and full of anticipation.

reproach To address (someone) in such a way as to express disapproval or disappointment.

quirk A peculiar behavioral habit.

rally A motorsport event in which motor vehicles similar in series drive partly on unpaved roads in the terrain.

rebuke Express sharp disapproval or criticism of someone because of his or her behavior or actions.

reproach To address (someone) in such a way as to express disapproval or disappointment.

rhetoric The art of lecturing (effective or persuasive speaking or writing, especially the use of figures of speech and other compositional techniques).

Rorschach Psychological test in which inkblots are used to determine a person's personality, according to the Swiss Psychiatrist Herman Rorschach.

ruminate To think deeply about something.

run dry Cease to exist, vanish.

settlement An agreement by giving in to each other. The costs of the litigation are shared or determined by the judge. However, the plaintiff remains responsible for lawyer and court expenses if nothing can be obtained from the other side. In the case of a settlement, the lawyer earns more.

shard A piece of broken ceramic, metal, glass or rock, typically having sharp edges.

Shaw, George Bernard (1856-1950) An Irish playwright, critic, polemicist and political activist.

speck Smoked or pickled pork belly. In Germany, speck is pork fat with or without some meat in it.

stamp out To end it.

STD Also known as sexually transmitted infection or STI; transmitted through sexual contact; caused by bacteria, viruses or parasites.

subtle Especially of a change or distinction. So delicate or precise as to be difficult to analyze or describe.

symbiont Symbionts live in a symbiosis in which coexistence exists for mutual benefit. Symbionts are the things or people that one needs to live. Planet Earth, with its ecological systems, is a symbiont for the human, whereby the human has to take care of the maintenance of the system, otherwise he himself will perish.

thematic Having or relating to subjects or a particular subject. Belonging to, relating to, or denoting the theme of a sentence. A body of topics for study or discussion.

thetan [Greek, *theta* = spirit] A spiritual being.

training Teaching or developing in oneself or others any skills and knowledge or fitness that relate to specific useful competencies. Training has specific goals of improving one's capability, capacity, productivity and performance.

trait A distinguishing quality or characteristic, typically one belonging to a person.

treacherous Dangerous.

trichomoniasis Also called trich, is a sexually transmitted infection caused by a parasite. It is among the most common sexually transmitted infections. Risk factors include multiple sexual partners and not using condoms during sex. More than three million U.S. cases per year.

vernacular The language or dialect spoken by the ordinary people in a particular country or region.

vexation The state of being annoyed, frustrated or worried.

yogi A practitioner of yoga, including a sannyasin or practitioner of meditation.

Sources and References

[1] Ferreira Peter: Water & Salt, the Essence of Life: The Healing Power of Nature, Natural Health Intl, 1. November 2003

[2] Hubbard, L. Ron: Science of Survival, L.A. U.S.A: Bridge Publications Inc. 2007

[3] Diamond Harvey und Marilyn, Fit fürs Leben, Goldmann Verlag, 1. Februar 1990

[4] Hubbard, L. Ron: Dianetics – The Modern Science of Mental Health, L.A. U.S.A: Bridge Publications Inc. 2007

[5] Konz, Franz, Der große Konz ... 1000 ganz legale Steuertricks, Droemer Knaur, 2003

About the Author

I, Wolfgang Fries, was born in St. Wendel/Saarland, Germany, on January 16, 1966.

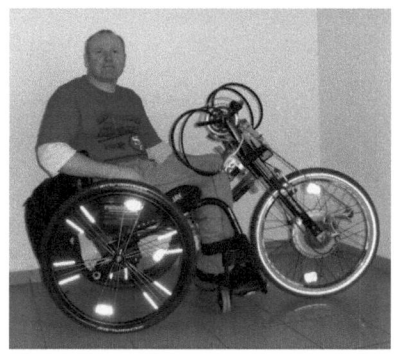

I had a standard education that included technical school. Afterward, I served five years in the Bundeswehr (German army) until 1994, when I started working as a stucco master, an occupation that enriched my life. I was easily able to form social contacts and was still well-liked after work. By forming a few friendships, I felt a social bond with others.

Unfortunately, I had to stop this nice work. As it turned out, bad things can lead to a good result. If I were not sitting in a wheelchair, I never would have written all of this. During a disastrous accident with the motorcycle, I broke my spine and since then have been permanently paralyzed.

But there is something in life everyone should know: Life itself. During all the work one does, and all the good times one enjoys, one should never forget this.

Exactly that was my endeavor.

It is not easy to find out what or who you are. If you're a tradesman, engineer, thinker, or racing professional. You can be anything you only have to decide!

My Philosophy

Life itself wants to live. All knowledge could be packed into a pyramid, where at the tip, only one word is present: life.

The word "life" by itself does not have enough meaning, and its definition does not give all the necessary information about its various types of existence.

Humanity has an abundance of knowledge, and yet we can detect that any doing or thinking can, in the end, be reduced to "life." Therefore, we have a hierarchy of importance.

Life will probably only be completely understood once all information has been collected, then evaluated, and associated – an impossible task, due to continuous creation of new knowledge and discoveries, and changes in perspectives, which require information to be evaluated and associated again. Perhaps a few main points will suffice to have orientation in life, and any knowledge regarding these main points can be expanded or replaced without changing the quality in understanding life significantly.

My Philosophy provides a few main points that are listed in the pyramid of knowledge directly below "life." The brief corollaries in My Philosophy may not be understood right away, and are the basis for the book Philosophy of Life, where life is addressed in more detail. It is like life itself, which can only be understood by having accumulated large amounts of information and personal experiences. The reader of My Philosophy will probably gain a deeper insight after having read Philosophy of Life and will therefore be able to compare and evaluate his personal experiences.

My Philosophy; 28 pages, 2018
ISBN: **978-3752892345**

What it Means to Be Human

What is a Human? Is it, as science wants you to believe, a creature that arose from mud or, as the priest tells you, a being of soul-motivated flesh? What and who are you? One thing for sure, dead matter doesn't think!

In this book, Wolfgang Fries critically examines the age-old philosophical question of what it means to be human using straight talk and common sense.

One thing is certain. You are alive and try to live a life as a human being. You have your notions of how to live your life, but your ideas regarding life are countered by certain intentions, which make life a difficult and complicated task. So we have these two things, your notions and counter intentions, which give you a frame of living. To subsist in life, a certain amount of knowledge and understanding is necessary. But to establish understanding, knowledge has to be evaluated with respect to right and wrong, important and unimportant.

The author maintains that only by understanding the complex issues that present themselves today will the human being be able to achieve personal goals and survive in this world. He covers such timely topics as coping with stress, fake news, the influence of the media, big pharma, big government, rampant materialism, illnesses and the novel coronavirus. No prior knowledge of moral philosophy is necessary to benefit from what readers will surely find to be an indispensable book.

What it Means to Be Human; 204 pages, 2020
ISBN: **978-3-7526-4352-7**

Human Rights and Obligations - Revised

The assurance of human rights in an orderly environment is the foundation for a peaceful existence and a thriving civilization. In a hostile environment with fighting and destruction, there is no peaceful existence, and a civilization cannot prosper through achievements in medicine, technology and science, all of which contribute to the welfare of humanity.

But what distinguishes human rights, so that there can be a peaceful coexistence that contributes to the welfare of humans?

First, humans need the basic attitude followed by the corresponding knowledge and a code to achieve this, thus, making it something that everyone must work on.

Human Rights and Obligations - Revised; 36 pages, 2018
ISBN: **978-3748130062**

An Ace at the Nürburgring-Nordschleife - Handbook -

What top speed is possible at each spot?

The handbook with more than 130 photographs and 26 sketches of each section of the track; and a max speed during good weather conditions with Bridgestone BT 56/57 tires on a Yamaha FZR 1000. Track time 8.06 minutes. "He who knows danger can face it!"

An Ace at the Nürburgring-Nordschleife - Handbook -; 80 pages, 2018
ISBN: **978-3-7528-6921-7**

Philosophie des Lebens - Das Buch der Grundlagen -

Was sind die Grundlagen des Daseins? Welche Geisteshaltung bedarf es in der heutigen Zeit um im Leben bestehen zu können, um Glück und Wohlergehen zu erfahren? Was ist wichtig zu wissen?

Der Mensch selbst, als denkendes Wesen ist der Ansicht, dass seine mächtigste Waffe der Verstand ist. Aufgrund seiner Fähigkeit zu denken hat er sich die Erde zum Untertan gemacht. Und tatsächlich, das Denken bestimmt das Handeln des Menschen, der Mensch ist nur so stabil wie sein Gedanke.

Der Gedanke selbst fußt auf Grundlagen die bestimmend dazu sind, wie man überlebt. So versucht der Mensch sich selbst, sein Denken und Handeln, die Welt um sich herum zu verstehen.

Verstehen: Was ist wichtiger als Verstehen selbst?

Grundlagen komprimiert verpackt, in kurzen Texten dargestellt. Mehr als 200 Essays führen den Leser zu mehr Verstehen im Leben und über das Leben selbst, sei es nun über den Menschen, das Denken, Glücklichsein, Beziehung, Lernen, Beruf, den Ursprung von Krankheiten, gesellschaftliches Dasein, Religion, Politik oder Freiheit.

Die Probleme des Menschen werden von der Ursache her geschildert und Lösungen angeboten. Es macht einen Unterschied dieses Wissen zu haben und sich dadurch selbst zu helfen.

Als Taschenbuch oder als Bibliotheken-Ausgabe im extra stabilen Hardcover-Format und Fadenbindung herausgegeben. *Philosophie des Lebens – Das Buch der Grundlagen* ist der Gesamt-Band welcher die Bücher *Meine Philosophie, Lernen wie man lernt, lernen wie man versteht, Eine glückliche Beziehung führen, Rückführung – Einführung und Kurzanleitung* und ehemals *Im Leben bestehen – Die Bibel des 21sten Jahrhunderts* in einem Buch vereint.

Philosophie des Lebens - Das Buch der Grundlagen -; 656 Seiten, 2017.

ISBN: **978-3-7357-8561-9** - Hardcover,

ISBN: **978-3-7460-2923-8** - Taschenbuch

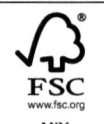